THE HEART-LUNG MACHINE
&
RELATED TECHNOLOGIES
OF
OPEN HEART SURGERY

By

Jon W. Austin, C.C.P.
David L. Harner

Written and produced with the cooperation and assistance
of
St. Luke's Medical Center's Heart Lung Center
Phoenix, Arizona

Phoenix Medical Communication
Medical Publishers
Phoenix, Arizona

The Heart Lung Machine
&
Related Technologies of Open Heart Surgery.

By Jon W. Austin and David L. Harner.

Phoenix Medical Communication.
Phoenix, Arizona.

Second Printing 1990

Library of Congress Catalog Card Number 89-091429
ISBN 0-938633-00-7

Printed and bound in the United States of America
at
Arrowhead Press, Inc.
Phoenix, Arizona

Dedication

To Our Wives

Kathie Austin and Carol Harner

ACKNOWLEDGEMENTS

The authors gratefully acknowledge...

The editorial assistance of:
Rebecca Kuhn, R.N., M.S.N.
Tim Thieroff, C.C.P.
Angelos K.Iatridis, C.C.P.

The artistic talent of Charles A. Arquette, Scottsdale, Arizona.

The contributions and advice of:
Mark Kartub, M.D.
E. Lawrence Ganter, M.D.
Cecil C. Vaughn, M.D.

The assistance of Kay Wellik, Medical Librarian, Phoenix, Arizona.

The biomedical manufacturing companies who provided photos and illustrations of their products.

The Heart Lung Center of St. Luke's Medical Center, Phoenix, Arizona for its encouragement and assistance with the book's illustration.

Our families, who spent many hours without us as a result of our labors.

The Authors

PREFACE

Our intention in writing this book is not to create an exhaustive tome about the heart-lung machine; our intention is to create a brief overview about the technologies of open-heart surgery.

This work may suffice for some, such as the student who has a casual interest in cardiovascular medicine, the health care professional who has a modest interest in open heart surgery, or the knowledgeable layman who needs basic information for a research or writing project. For others, such as the professional associated with open heart surgery and the student of cardiovascular perfusion, we hope that this book will be a place to begin—a précis, if you will, that will stimulate and direct further study.

Cardiovascular perfusion (operation of the heart-lung machine) is not an exact science, but rather an art. The thousands of perfusionists who successfully operate heart-lung machines all over the world operate them with slightly varying techniques. It is our hope that these differences in technique will serve as stimuli for further discussion. Therefore, the opinions concerning perfusion techniques should not be accepted as the only opinions, nor necessarily the definitive ones.

Jon Austin, C.C.P.
David L. Harner

TABLE OF CONTENTS

Section III: Techniques & Problems

SECTION I

INTRODUCTION

CHAPTER ONE

Before medical professionals could devise an artificial circulation, they first had to make a detailed description of the natural circulation. This description took scientists several centuries. (Figure 1.1)

One of the Greek scientists, Galen, born in 131 A.D., was a noted philosopher, writer, and physician. From his experience in the dissection of animals, such as sheep, oxen, dogs, bears, and apes, Galen wrote a text entitled, *In Preparatio Collegium (On Anatomical Preparations)*. It became the standard medical textbook for some fourteen hundred years—probably the longest time that any such textbook enjoyed popularity in the scientific community.

Galen deduced that blood in the circulatory system was produced in the liver (then thought to be the seat of man's passions) and carried to the heart. Once in the heart, Galen thought, the blood passed from the right heart to the left heart through pores in the septum. The blood, after passage through the heart, then became mixed with air in the lungs. Galen believed that a "boiling up" or "fermenting" process heated the body and instilled a motion in the blood that carried it to all the body parts. He supposed that the blood pumped from the heart was "used up" by the body and never returned.

Galen's description of the circulation was irrefutable from his death about 200 A.D. until William Harvey's demonstration of continous circulation in the seventeenth century. Many of Galen's thoughts and descriptions about the circulation of the blood were based on the philosophical writings of Aristotle and Plato.

William Harvey (1578-1657) was an Englishman

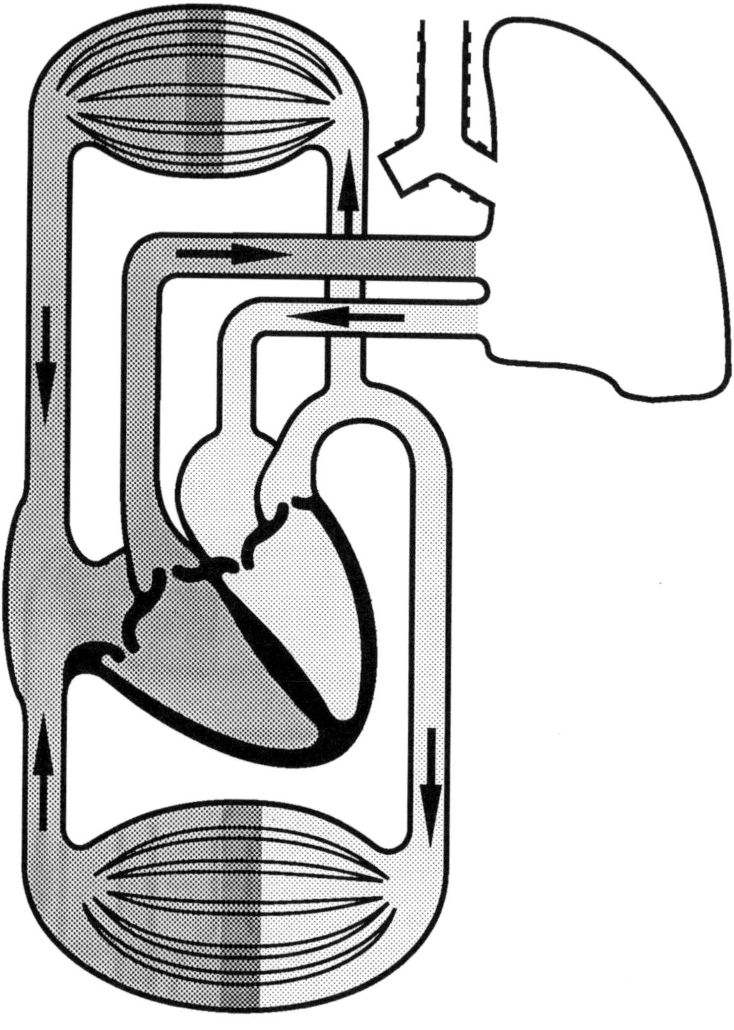

Normal Circulation

Figure 1.1 It took scientists several centuries to describe adequately the natural circulation.

who obtained his early medical education at the University of Padua in Italy (Figure 1.2). He was widely-respected—so much so that he became the private physician to King James I. In addition to his medical practice, Harvey was a skilled student of human anatomy who published his findings. The work that brought him the most fame was the book *De Motu Cordis (The Beating Heart)* (Figure 1.3). In several experiments, Harvey measured the amount of blood leaving the heart and concluded that it was quite impossible for the body to manufacture as much blood as thought by Galen. Although he apparently did not see the capillaries that we know connect the arteries with the veins, he postulated that there must be some kind of connection between the two structures.

As early as 1812, a French physician, Julien-Jean Cesar LeGallois, proposed the idea of artificial circulation. He suggested that the heart could be replaced by a pump that would supply *arterial* blood to keep any isolated part of the body alive for an indefinite time. His experiments attempted to perfuse the bodies of decapitated rabbits by injection, but the experiments proved inconclusive.

Two German researchers, Ludwig and Schmidt, first artificially oxygenated blood in 1869. They took defibrinated blood and simply shook it along with gas in a balloon.

During the next 75 years, other scientists, most of them German, worked to develop ways of oxygenating the blood. Von Schroeder was credited with the introduction of the first bubble oxygenator in 1882. Three years later, von Frey and Gruber introduced the first film oxygenator, a refined device by which blood could be oxygenated by filming it over a rotating cylinder without interrupting blood flow.

There were many other experimenters and devices—oxygenators, pumps, and driving systems. For example, a perfusion apparatus which "permitted an entire organ to live outside the body" was proposed in 1935 by Alexis Carrel and Charles A. Lindbergh, the famous aviator. A man of

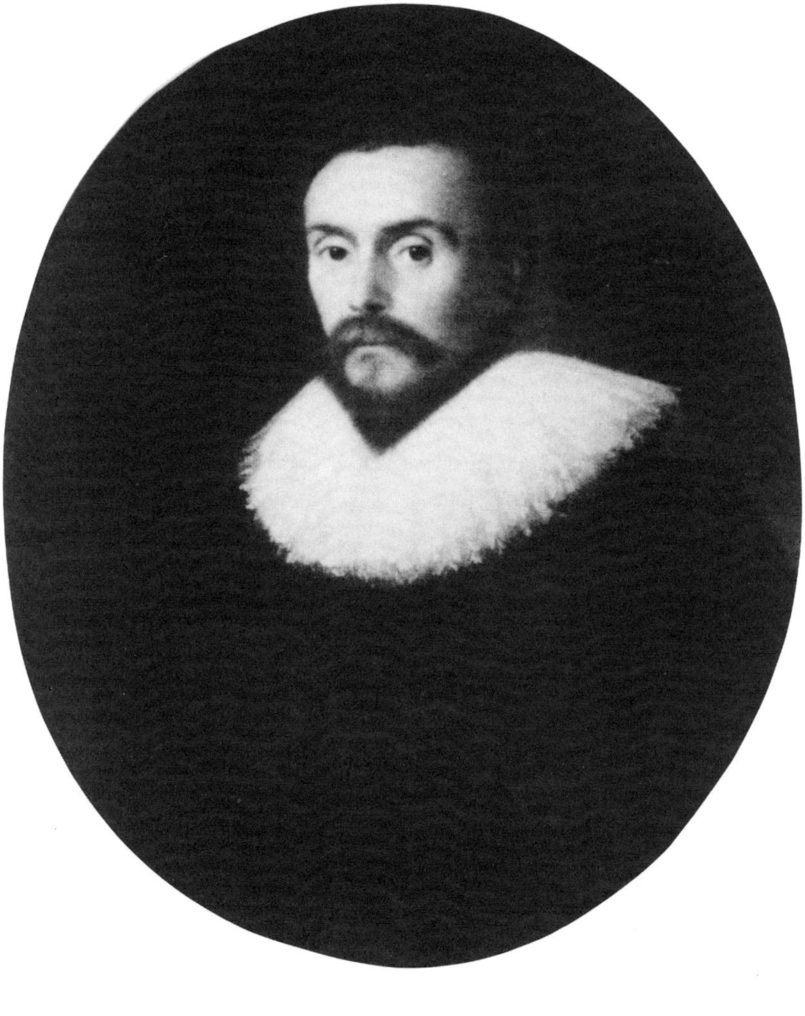

Figure 1.2 Known as "Father of Modern Circulation," William Harvey established the foundation for today's knowledge of the human circulatory system.

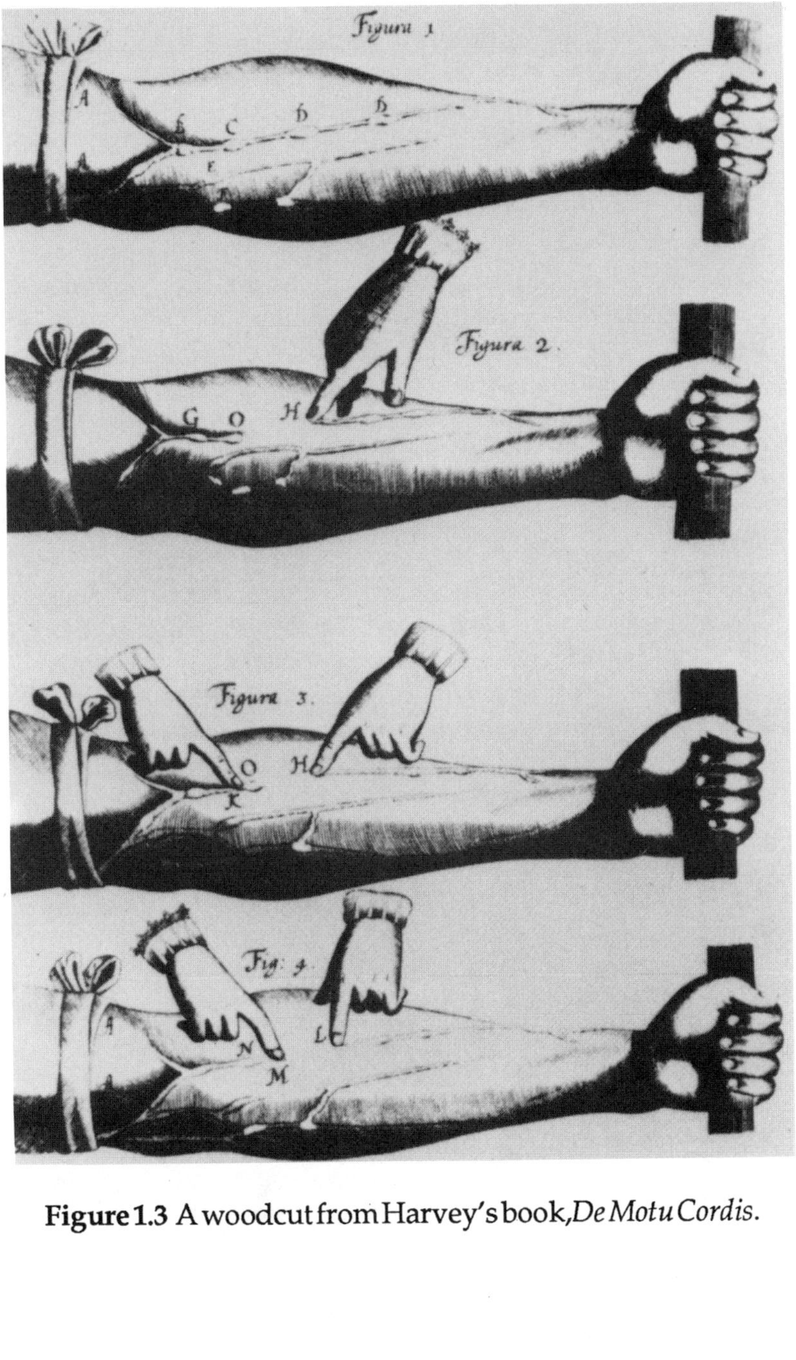

Figure 1.3 A woodcut from Harvey's book, *De Motu Cordis.*

many interests, Lindbergh had become a biochemical assistant to Carrel at the Rockefeller Institute.

The next major development in artificial perfusion, however, had its origins a few years earlier, in 1931. A young surgeon, Dr. John H. Gibbon, Jr., was assisting an operating team at Massachusetts General Hospital. A female patient had suffered a massive postoperative pulmonary embolism. In the operating room, Dr. Gibbon's assignment was to watch the patient and take vital signs through the night. The surgical team waited to operate until it appeared that the patient would otherwise die. In those days, the risk of such a procedure (pulmonary embolectomy) was so great that operating before the patient was actually dying was to take an unjustified risk.

(From the "Recollections" of Mary Gibbon, Dr. Gibbon's wife): *During the hours that night that Jack watched the patient's distended veins and recorded the faltering pulse, respirations, and blood pressure, the thought occurred and constantly recurred to him that her condition could surely be improved if only there were some way of continuously withdrawing some of the blue blood from the swollen veins into an apparatus where the blood could pick up oxygen and discharge carbon dioxide, and then be pumped back into the patient's arteries.*

After the six and one-half minute operation, the patient did not survive. Yet the idea did survive in Dr. Gibbon's mind that such a machine could be designed.

In subsequent animal experiments in a one-room laboratory at Massachusetts General, Dr. Gibbon, assisted by his wife, did design an apparatus which he described in an article published in the *Archives of Surgery* in 1937. His machine, a vertical rotating cylinder that filmed blood to oxygenate it, along with a modified pump to maintain circulation, permitted bypass of the heart and lungs in experimental animals. This advancement from the perfusion of isolated organs to total body perfusion was moved forward rapidly by the discovery and availability of heparin, which prevented clotting. Gibbon's contribution is described as "perhaps the most important single development in the history of extracorporeal circulation." (However, one might also say that the discovery of heparin paralleled the importance of Gibbon's work.) Later experiments at the University of Pennsylvania Medical School and at the Jefferson Medical College in Philadelphia enabled Dr. Gibbon to perfect his machine. Dr. Gibbon's experiments were temporarily halted by World War II, during which he served as an armed forces surgeon.

On May 6, 1953, Dr. Gibbon began a new era of cardiac surgery when he successfully closed an atrial-septal defect in an eighteen year old girl using a heart-lung machine. It was the first such operation in the world.

Dr. Gibbon's "machine" helped usher in modern open heart surgery as we now know it. Since that time, hundreds of thousands of people have undergone open heart surgery with the use of the heart-lung machine. Because of it, the cardiovascular surgeon can operate on a heart under direct vision, in a relatively dry, relatively still operative field (Figure 1.4).

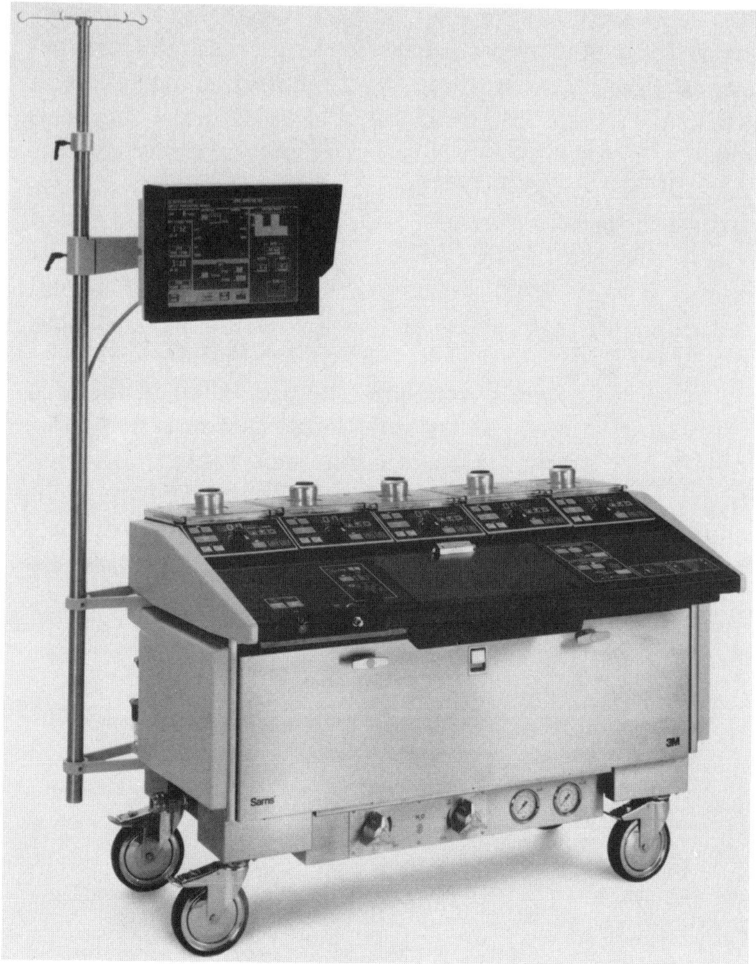

Figure 1.4 Modern heart-lung machines are both sophisticated and highly reliable. (Courtesy of Sarns, 3M Healthcare, Ann Arbor, Michigan.)

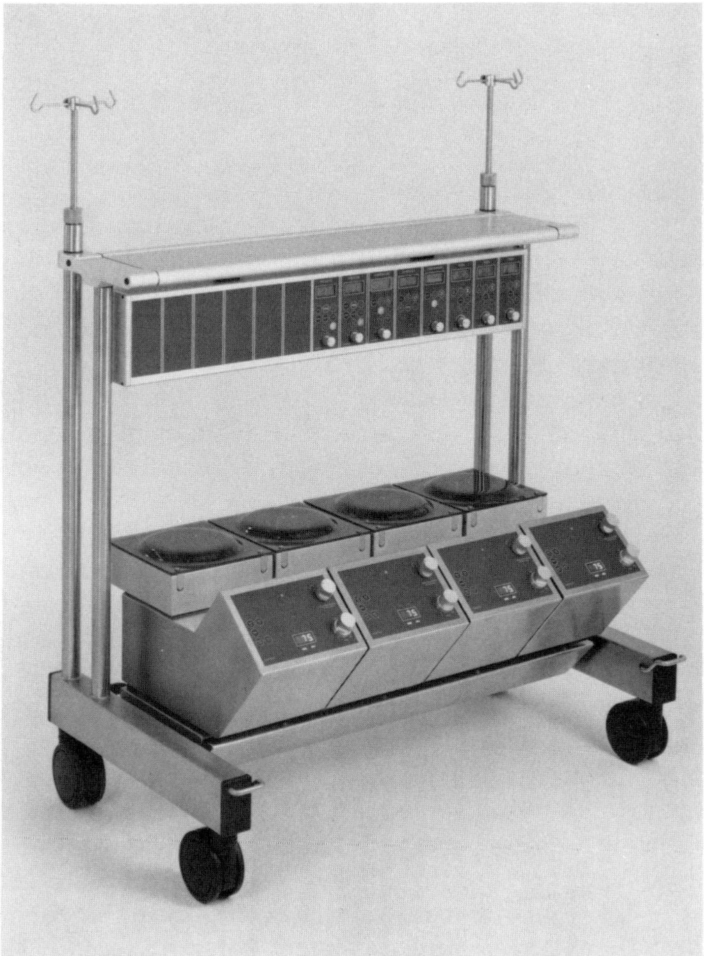

Figure 1.5 This heart-lung machine has a modular monitoring system and modular roller-type blood pumps. (Courtesy of Vitalcor, Inc. (Polystan), Westmont, Illinois.)

THE PRINCIPLES

Chapter Two

The Chemical Plant

Our bodies, in a sense, are little more than complex chemical plants. Modern heart-lung machines are nothing more than artificial chemical plants in which blood is continually processed. (Figure 2.1). Oxygen is added to the blood; carbon dioxide is removed. The oxygenated blood is pumped to the circulatory system and distributed in such a fashion that cellular metabolism can continue without interruption. Let's compare this process as it occurs naturally, with how it occurs in the heart-lung machine.

In nature, deoxygenated blood from the veins returns to the heart's right atrium (Figure 2.2). From the right atrium, blood is pumped to the right ventricle, then through the pulmonary artery to the lungs. The natural lung adds oxygen and removes carbon dioxide from the blood as it passes through the alveolar capillary network. After oxygenation, the blood is returned to the left atrium by way of the four pulmonary veins (Figure 2.3). Blood is then pumped through the mitral valve into the left ventricle, the main pumping chamber of the heart. As the left ventricle contracts, blood is pumped back into the systemic circulation. Oxygen is given up and carbon dioxide taken on as the blood passes through the body's capillary system. After this second gaseous exchange, the blood is returned to the right heart and the cycle is repeated.

During heart-lung bypass, venous blood is taken from the circulation by means of cannulae placed in the superior ad inferior vena cavae. The blood "bypasses" the heart and lungs and enters the machine's circuit (Figure 2.4). At this point, the circulation becomes "extracorporeal." It is

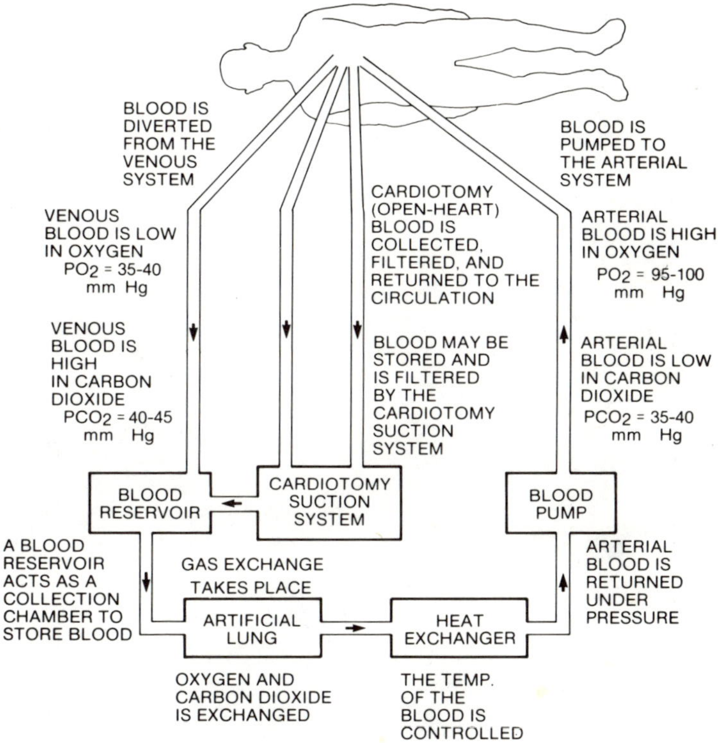

THE HEART-LUNG MACHINE IS LIKE A CHEMICAL PLANT

Figure 2.1

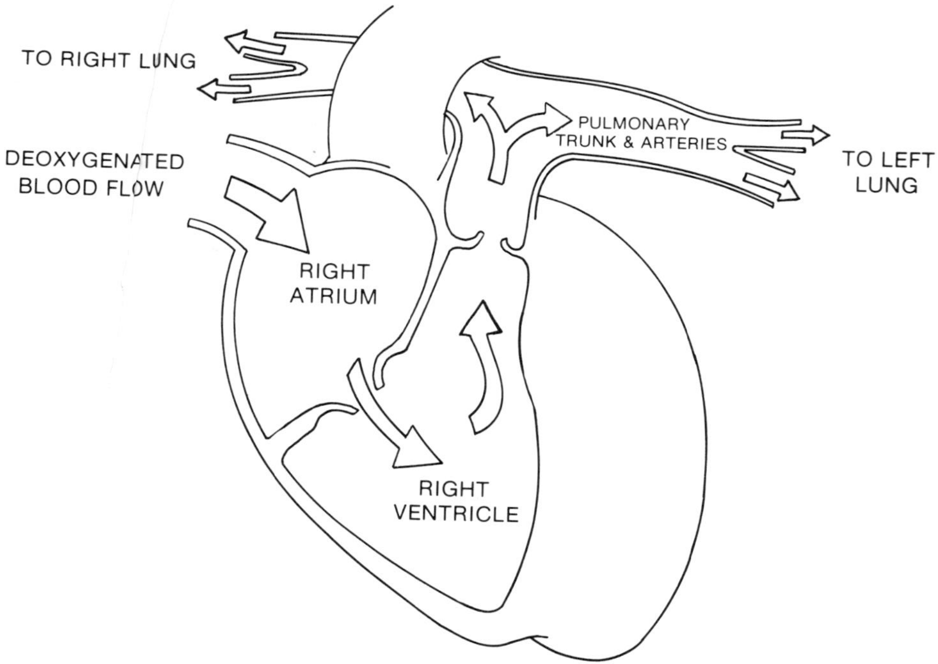

Figure 2.2 The right side of the heart pumps blood to the lungs where gas exchange takes place.

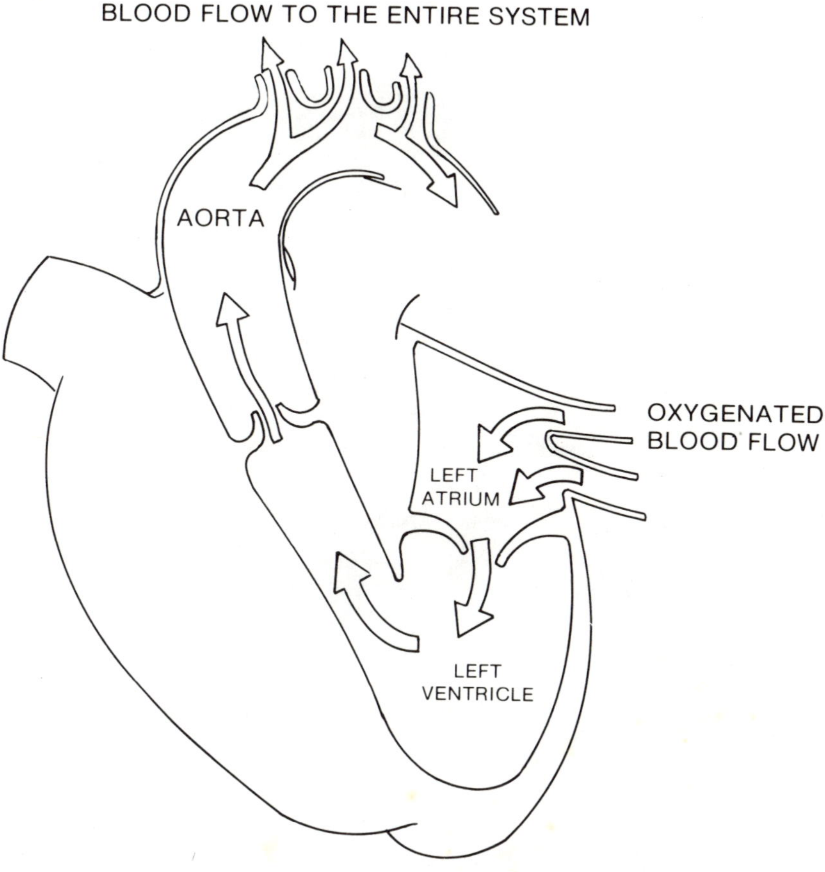

Figure 2.3 The left side of the heart pumps oxygenated blood to the systemic circulation.

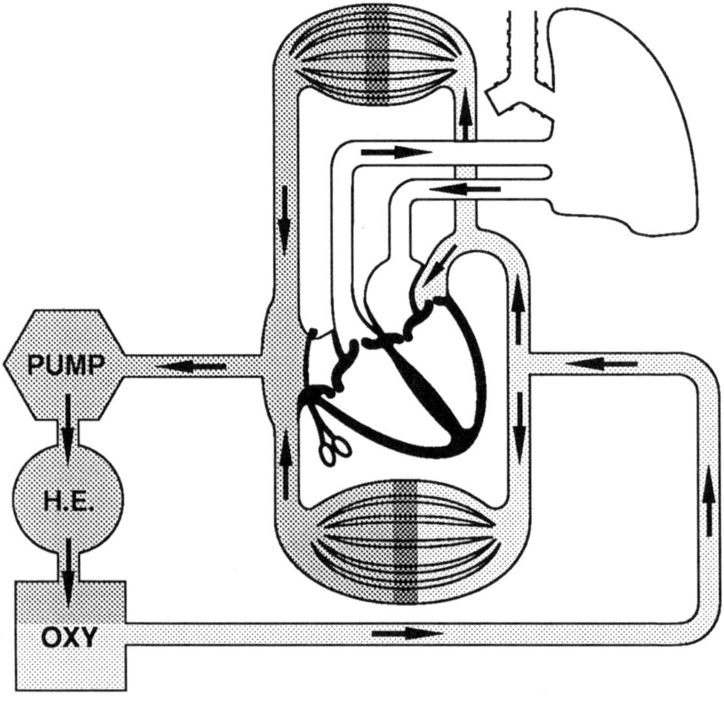

Total Cardiopulmonary Bypass

Figure 2.4 During heart-lung bypass, the blood is literally taken outside the body (extracorpareal) where heat exchange and gas exchange take place.

literally "outside the body." Oxygenation takes place in the machine's oxygenator or artificial lung much as it does in the natural process. The term "artificial lung" is perhaps more accurate since the device not only oxygenates the blood but also removes carbon dioxide. The artificial lung must remove carbon dioxide in the correct proportions to avoid excessive accumulation (causing respiratory acidosis) or excessive elimination (causing respiratory alkalosis). After being oxygenated, filtered, and temperature regulated, the blood is returned to the body's arterial circulation through a cannula.

Cardio-Respiratory Need

Individual cells, the building blocks of our bodies, require energy to carry on their functions. It is the job of the cardiovascular system to furnish the cells with their energy needs (Figure 2.5). This energy is supplied by foodstuffs that normally are metabolized in the presence of oxygen. Foodstuffs are carried to body cells in the blood plasma; oxygen is carried in the hemoglobin of the erythrocytes (as oxyhemoglobin) and in the plasma. As cellular metabolism occurs, a waste product is created—a gas, carbon dioxide (Figure 2.6). The carbon dioxide is carried in the form of carbonic acid ($H_2O + CO_2 \rightarrow H_2CO_3$) in both red cells and plasma to the lungs, where it is released in the form of a gas. The organic catalyst that triggers this transfer is an enzyme called "carbonic anahydrase." This description of oxygen and particularly carbon dioxide transfer is vastly simplified. A more complete description of these processes may be found in *The ABC of Acid-Base Chemistry* by Horace W. Davenport.

Total Metabolic Need

The basic metabolic needs of the body can best be equated in terms of total blood flow—the vehicle of body metabolism. If blood flow is reduced from its normal level, inadequate cellular metabolism results. Cells are capable, however, at least for a short time, of undergoing anaerobic metabolism—that is, metabolism without the presence of

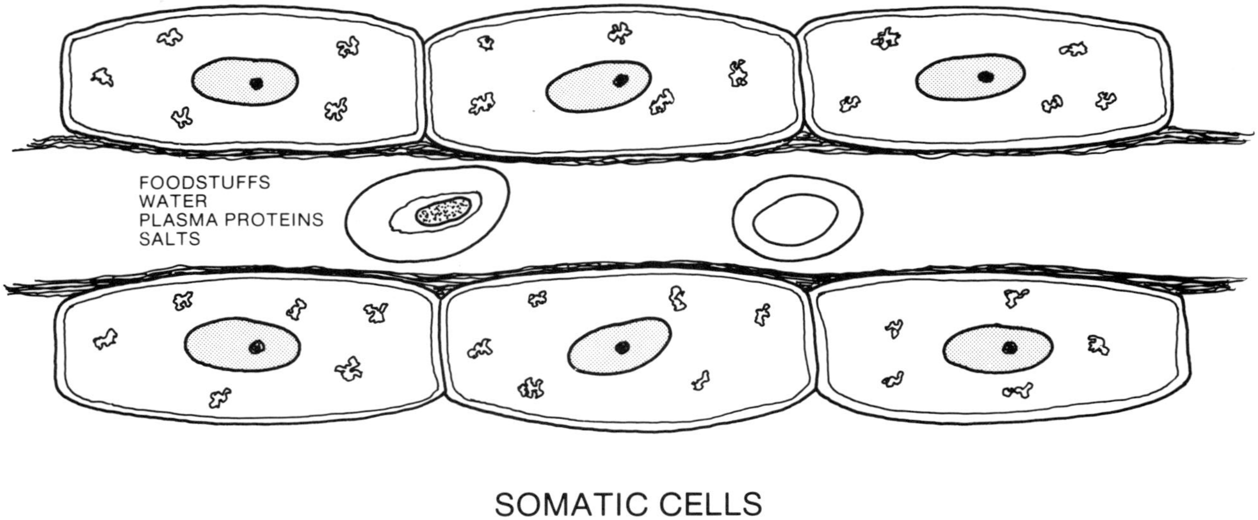

Figure 2.5 The cardiovascular system provides the somatic cells (all body cells that compose tissue and organs, excluding reproductive cells) with their chemical needs and removes their waste products.

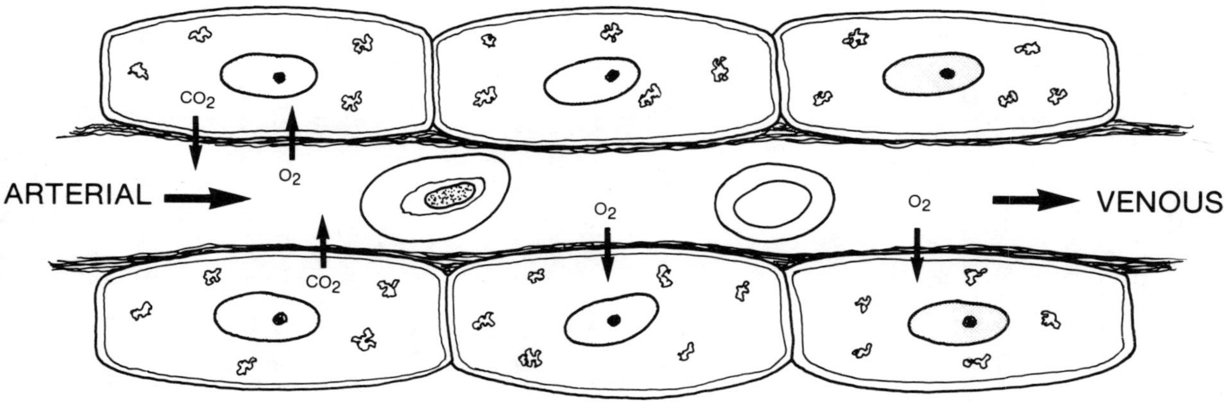

CELLULAR GAS EXCHANGE

Figure 2.6 Respiration involves gas exchange at the cellular level.

length of time that it takes body cells to use up their energy stores. A noteworthy by-product of anaerobic metabolism is lactic acid. An exhausted long-distance runner, for example, may experience anaerobic metabolism in muscle cells that are energy-depleted and in oxygen debt. As a result, there may be an excessive build-up of lactic acid in muscle cells. The runner may experience severe muscle cramps and other symptoms as a result of this state of lactic acidosis. During anaerobic metabolism, more acid accumulates than during normal metabolism. As a result, one may determine whether the blood flow is adequate during heart-lung bypass by monitoring the patient's acid-base balance. Inadequate blood flow is generally indicated by a lowered pH of the blood (higher acid level).

Protective Redistribution

The body has its own protective mechanism to maintain proper cellular metabolism. If total blood flow is reduced, say in the case of severe trauma or in heart-lung bypass, the body initiates a process called, "protective redistribution." During protective distribution, vital tissues of the body (such as brain, heart, kidneys, and viscera) receive more blood flow than less vital tissues (such as arms, legs, and skin). This process can take place for a limited amount of time while body processes (blood clotting, etc.) attempt to shore up the damage. Protective redistribution is caused primarily by changes in the vascular resistance produced by vasomotor activity in organ systems. In other words, blood vessels in high priority organs increase in size to enhance blood flow; blood vessels in low priority organs decrease in size to reduce blood flow.

In low flow perfusion, acid blood levels tend to increase (metabolic acidosis). Administration of sodium bicarbonate may be required to buffer the blood (raise the pH—lower the acid).

Total blood flow rates of a surgical patient with normal body temperature may be moderately reduced during perfusion because of the resting, anesthetized state.

The range of reduction allowed by this resting state is from 2.2 to 2.5 liters per square meter of body surface per minute. A normal cardiac index is approximately 3.5 liters per square meter of body surface per minute. Total human body surface may be calculated by a formula developed by DuBois (Figure 2.7).

Blood Flow During Hypothermia

Further reduction in blood flow while still maintaining adequate perfusion may be accomplished by lowering the patient's body temperature (hypothermia). Hypothermia lowers the body's metabolic rate, thus reducing oxygen demand. One may recall the instance in January of 1984 when a child fell into the 32° F waters of ice-covered Lake Michigan in the Chicago area. Although submerged for twenty minutes, the child made a complete physical recovery with only minimal brain damage because of severe hypothermia. The metabolic processes were so diminished, the oxygen demand so small, that survival was possible. Clinical hypothermia affords a safety margin for the patient should the heart-lung machine malfunction or should there be an unforseen problem with the surgical procedure.

Hypothermia produced by cooling the body's surface was employed in heart surgery before the advent of the heart-lung machine for the surgical treatment of uncomplicated atrial septal defects.

As a "rule of thumb," it can be stated that for each degree Centigrade that body temperature can be lowered, the metabolic demand of the body is lowered by approximately 7%. Thus, if a patient is cooled from normal temperature (37° C) to 30° C, the metabolic demand (oxygen utilization) is reduced by approximately 49%. "Deep hypothermia," the technique of lowering the core temperature of a patient below 20° C, allows a surgical team to stop circulation completely for a period of time (circulatory arrest), possibly up to one hour, but preferably limited to a few minutes.

Selective hypothermia may be used to protect vari-

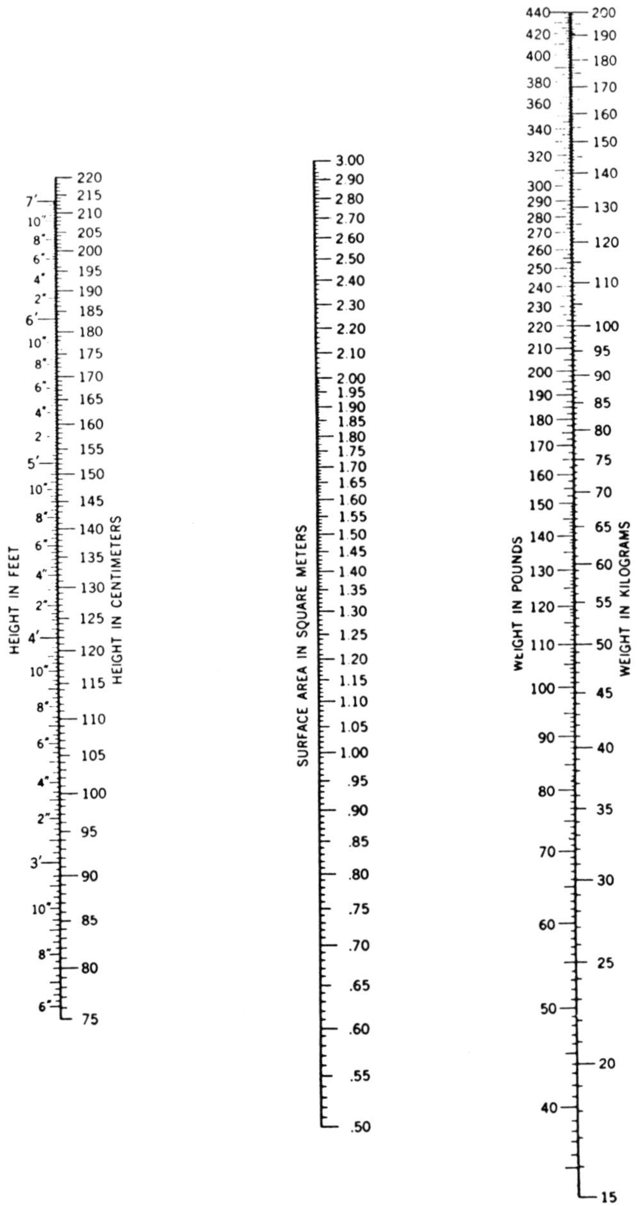

Figure 2.7 The Dubois body surface area normogram. See Appendix for formula.

ous organs during open heart surgery and during heart, kidney, and liver transplantations. During open heart surgery, the heart is often cooled during the operation by the injection of a cold fluid that is high in potassium directly into the coronary arteries. The injection causes the heart to stop, and the patient's body is supported on cardiopulmonary bypass. This technique is called "hypothermic cardioplegia" (literally, "paralysis of the heart caused by lowered temperature"). Hypothermic cardioplegia protects the heart during the period of myocardial ischemia, when the heart muscle has a decreased or nonexistent blood supply. Hypothermia is usually induced by means of a blood heat exchanger.

While less oxygen is used by the body and less carbon dioxide is produced as a product of metabolism during hypothermia, the process does create some problems. The solubility of both oxygen and carbon dioxide is increased at lower temperatures, and oxygen is more tightly bound by the oxyhemoglobin molecule. The interpretation of acid base balance during hypothermia is more complicated. Not all of the body tissues receive the same amount of blood flow, and there are many temperature gradients among the various organ systems during both cooling and rewarming of the body during the surgical procedure. During hypothermic perfusion, there may be a harmful condition involving a low partial pressure of carbon dioxide and an elevated blood pH (higher alkalinity) caused by the rapid drop in body temperature. For this reason, many perfusion teams choose to ventilate the artificial lung with carbon dioxide in an attempt to maintain a "normal" partial pressure of CO_2. However, other perfusion teams purposely ventilate with pure oxygen to lower the PCO_2 (a technique derived from the observation of hibernating animals, who under hypothermic conditions, maintain their CO_2 at lower levels).

It is beyond the scope of this book to describe all the acid base changes which may take place during hypothermia. At this point in the state-of-the-art, all of the body's physiologic parameters during hypothermia are not known.

DYNAMIC EQUILIBRIUM

CHAPTER THREE

The Fluid Compartment

Water composes a large part of our bodies. Water in the form of *intra*cellular fluid is found within cell membranes. Water in the form of *extra*cellular fluid is found outside of the cell in all body tissues. Extracellular fluid can be further defined as "intravascular" and "interstitial" (Figure 3.1). Intravascular fluid is contained within the blood vessels and the heart (the intravascular space). Interstitial fluid fills the space between the capillary wall and the cell membrane. It is in this space that the exchange (diffusion) of food stuffs, gases, and chemical waste products must take place. Because of injury or disease, at times this interstitial space may become "engorged" or filled with fluid. This condition is known as "edema" or "third spacing."

The chemical composition of the fluids in each of the fluid spaces must be maintained within rather narrow limits for everything to work well. It is the constant movement of the heart which causes the continual flow of intravascular fluid. Intravascular fluid exchanges molecules and ions with the interstitial fluid, and interstitial fluid is exchanged with the intracellular fluid. This process is referred to as "dynamic equilibrium."

Among other functions, the blood and circulatory systems provide a method whereby specialized tissues can chemically communicate with the body cells to carry on body functions. For example, food is processed by the digestive system and converted into a form of chemical energy that is usable by the cells. This chemical energy is distributed to the cells by the blood. In another example, waste products are eliminated when products of cellular metabolism are transported by the blood to the kidneys,

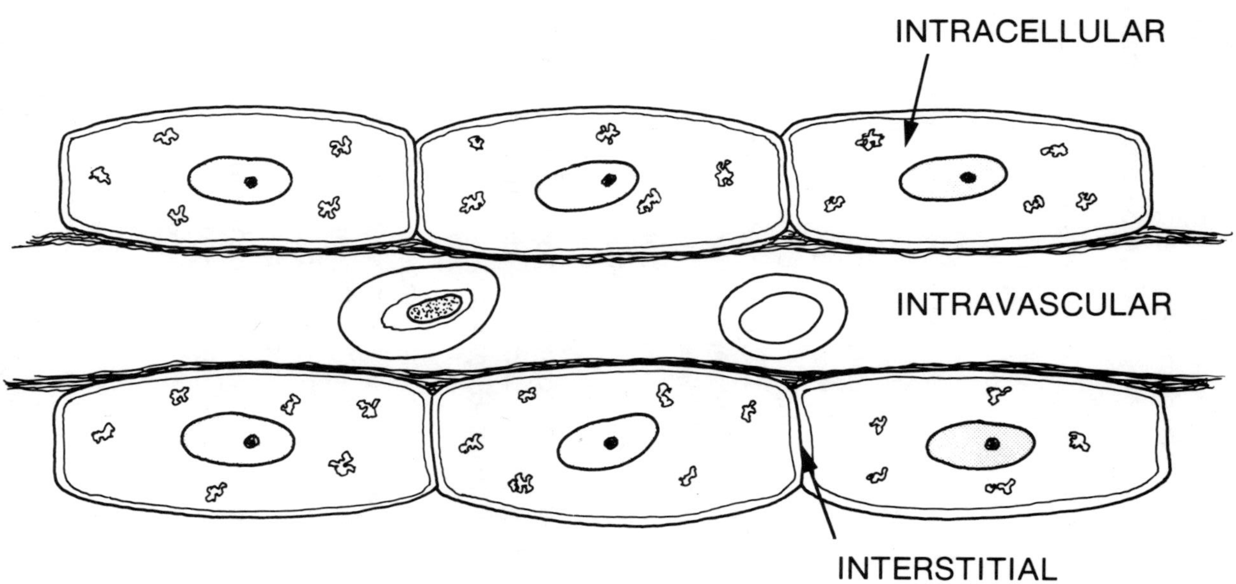

Figure 3.1 The fluid spaces.

converted to urine, and excreted. Epinephrine is manufactured by the adrenal glands and is not secreted directly into the blood stream, but rather is diffused into the blood through the interstitial spaces.

In all these necessary body functions, blood is the transportation system—propelled by the heart and carried to each individual cell by the blood vessels.

Transport

Diffusion:

At the capillary level, transportation of fluids through "fluid compartments" and membranes is regulated by natural physical laws. Molecules are constantly in motion, and they move in random directions. The speed in which molecules move is in direct proportion to their temperature—the higher the temperature of the molecules, the faster they will move If the molecular concentration of a substance varies from one part or region of the substance to another, there is a tendency for molecules in the area of greater concentration to move to an area of lesser concentration. This movement is called "diffusion." Solids and gases also move across cell membranes by diffusion (Figure 3.2).

Osmosis:

Water and other fluids move from a region of greater concentration to a region of lesser concentration across a semi-permeable membrane by the process of osmosis. Movement across the semi-permeable membrane is not only determined by the concentration gradient, but also by the degree of permeability of the membrane and by the molecular size and physical characteristics of the liquid crossing the membrane.

Cell Membranes:

Cell membranes are thought to be composed of layers of proteins and lipids. Membranes are perforated with water-filled pores. Water and smaller ions, such as potassium and chloride, can easily pass through the cell membrane pores. Cell membranes are obviously highly permeable to oxygen and carbon dioxide.

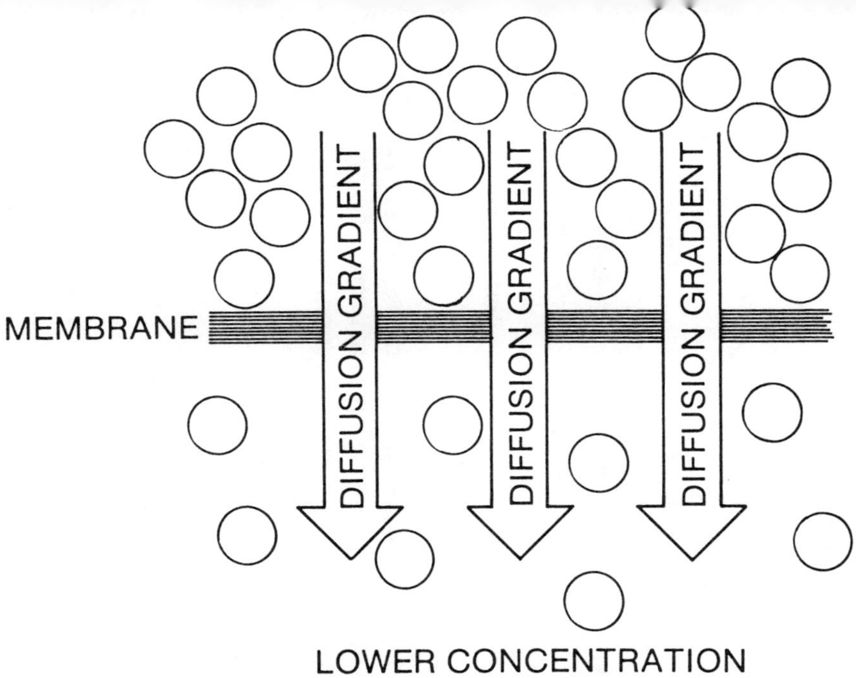

Figure 3.2 Diffusion takes place across a permeable membrane according to a diffusion gradient from a region of higher concentration to a region of lower concentration.

Pinocytosis:
Another way in which a substance can transverse a cell membrane is by a special lipid-soluble "carrier molecule." Certain ions can combine with the "carrier molecules" and be transported into the cell. This is how molecules too large to pass through openings in the cell membrane can get in and out of the cell.

The Blood

Most of us think of blood as a fluid. Although there is a fluid component of blood, it is more correct to think of blood as a collection of solids in a fluid suspension. The solids in suspension are its formed elements. If fresh, anticoagulated blood is collected in a test tube and centrifuged, several components become evident (Figure 3.3). At the top of the tube will be a straw-colored fluid—plasma. Upon close examination, the next component is a very thin layer of whitish material—the white blood cells and the platelets. The next component, the one that is obviously the most dense, is the red cells.

The laboratory process used to measure the cellular volume of a blood sample is called a "hematocrit." The word literally means "to separate blood." The volume of cells in a blood sample is expressed as a percentage. Normal hematocrit values vary from 38% to 54% of the total blood volume (see Appendix).

Let's return for a moment to the blood component at the top of the test tube—the plasma. Plasma is more than 90% water. The water acts as a solvent to carry nutritive materials, hormones, enzymes, and waste products. Plasma contains over 60 different plasma proteins. Plasma proteins are large molecules that are important in the regulation of optimal osmotic pressure gradients. In a simplistic way, this means that these proteins help to regulate the pressure on either side of the cell membrane so that chemical exchanges can take place.

White blood cells, or leukocytes, are somewhat larger than red cells (Figure 3.4). Unlike the immotile red blood

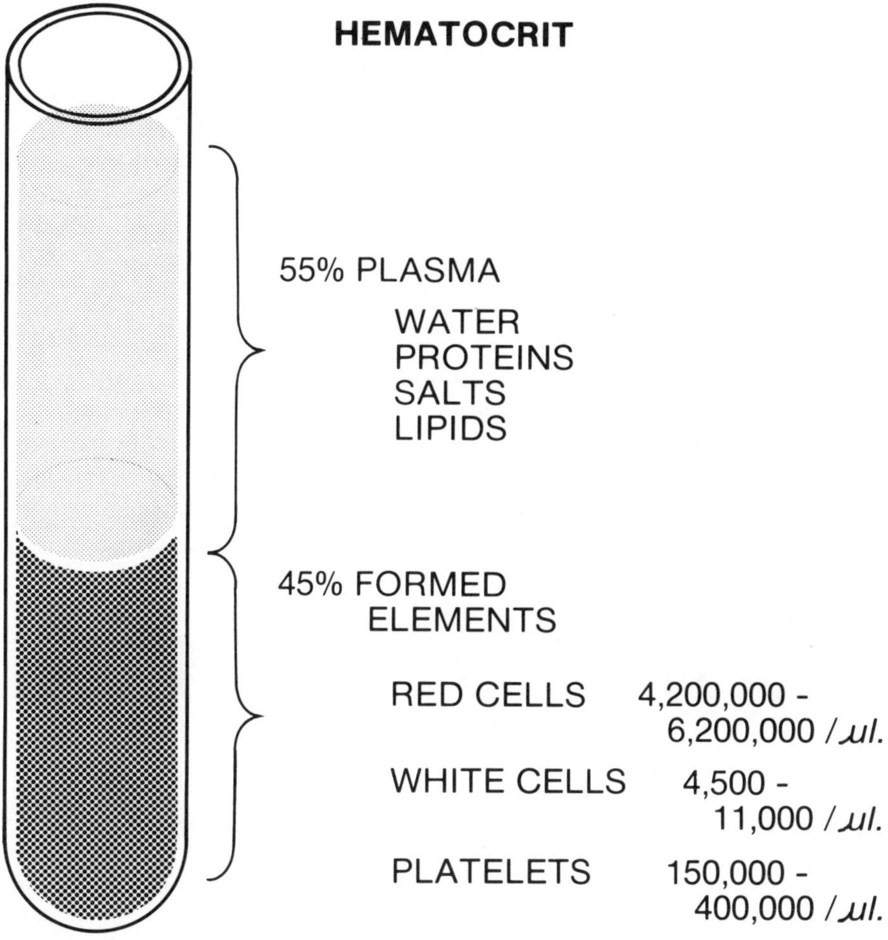

Figure 3.3 The centrifugation process allows one to separate the blood into its various components.

cells, white blood cells are capable of independent movement by amoeba-like action. They can change their shape and squeeze through the spaces between the endothelial cells of the capillary walls. They can also change shape to engulf bacterial cells (biochemically foreign material) and render them harmless by a process called "phagocytosis." *Phagein* is the Greek root for "to eat." White blood cells are attracted and stimulated to attack by chemical substances produced by bacterial cells. These substances, known as "toxins," are products of the bacterial cells' metabolic activity. This entire chemical system that stimulates the leukocytes is known as "the complement activation system." An additional task of the leukocytes is to destroy damaged or broken red blood cells. A normal white blood cell count is between 4,500-11,000 cells per microliter. Counts over this range may be indicative of an infection.

Small disks called "blood platelets" are the smallest cells found in the blood (Figure 3.4). Normal platelet counts range from 150,000 to 400,000 cells per microliter. Platelets, along with certain of the plasma proteins, are responsible for the action of forming networks of fibers that aid in the clotting process. Activation of the coagulation mechanism leads to a series of cascading chemical reactions which ultimately lead to blood coagulation.

Erythrocytes, or red blood cells, are biconcave disks which measure from 7-8 microns in diameter and are approximately 2.6 microns thick (Figure 3.4). Under a microscope they appear a pale copper color. When viewed in a test tube as a blood sample, however, they appear to be a brilliant red. The red color is mostly due to a protein—hemoglobin. Erythrocytes carry oxygen in the form of oxyhemoglobin to body cells and provide an enzyme, carbonic anahydrase, that controls the chemical reaction for carrying carbon dioxide. Every 100 milliliters of blood contains from 12 to 18 grams of hemoglobin. Each gram of hemoglobin can carry 1.34 milliliters of oxygen. Therefore, the normal oxygen-carrying capacity for each 100 milliliters of blood is from 16 to 24 milliliters of oxygen.

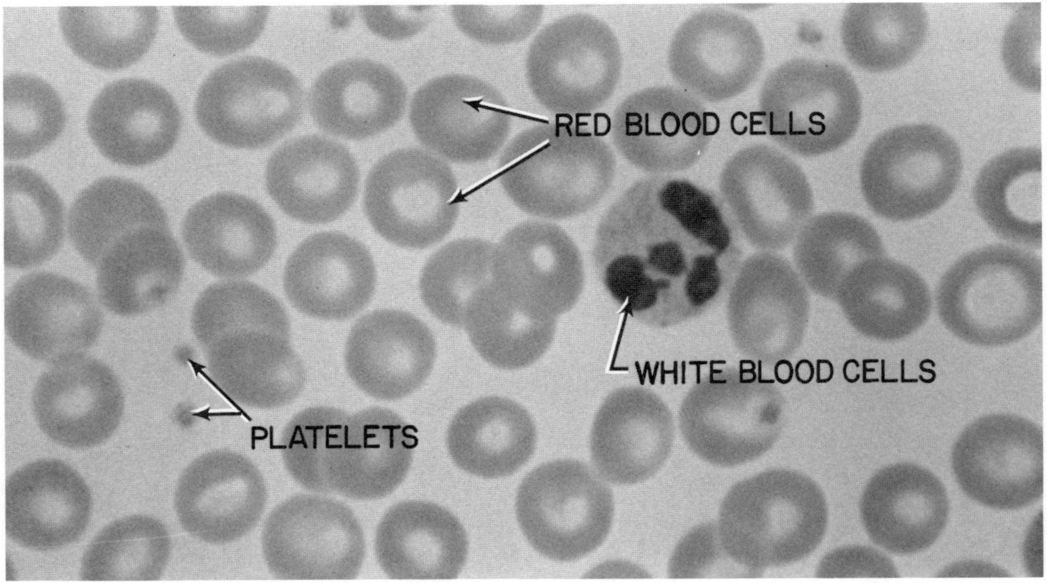

Figure 3.4 A white blood cell is seen surrounded by red blood cells and platelets. The dark spots are nuclei. (Courtesy of St. Luke's Medical Center's Patholgy Department, Phoenix, Arizona.)

Hematologic values depend upon a patient's age, sex, and state of health. (See the Appendix.)

SECTION II
COMPONENTS

THE PUMP

Chapter Four

The human heart is an ideal blood pump. The heart beats (pumps) 60-100 times per minute, 32,000,000-53,000,000 times during the course of a year. The human heart pumps 4 liters of blood (about 1 gallon) per minute—about 2,100,000 liters (about 520,000 gallons) per year in the "average" adult at rest. The fuel that powers this efficient pump can be derived from peaches or from pizza, from carrots or from candy bars. For all of its work and rigorous contractions, the heart handles blood in so gentle a fashion that its cellular elements are not damaged.

Types of Pumps

The human heart may be described mechanically as a reciprocating-type pump. Its pumping chambers are alternately filled and emptied by a very complex back and forth displacement of the ventricular walls. Its unidirectional flow is accomplished by propelling the blood through one-way valves located at the inlet and the outlet of the pumping chambers, the ventricles. All reciprocating-type pumps, including the human heart, produce a pulsatile flow (Figure 4.1).

Many reciprocating-type pumps have been used for artificial perfusion: the bellows-type, the piston-type, and the ventricle-sac-type. The ventricle-sac-type reciprocating pump (Figure 4.2) operates in a way that is very similar to the human heart. A ventricle-sac type pump was implanted in the chest of Dr. Barney Clark in 1983. Dr. Clark was the first

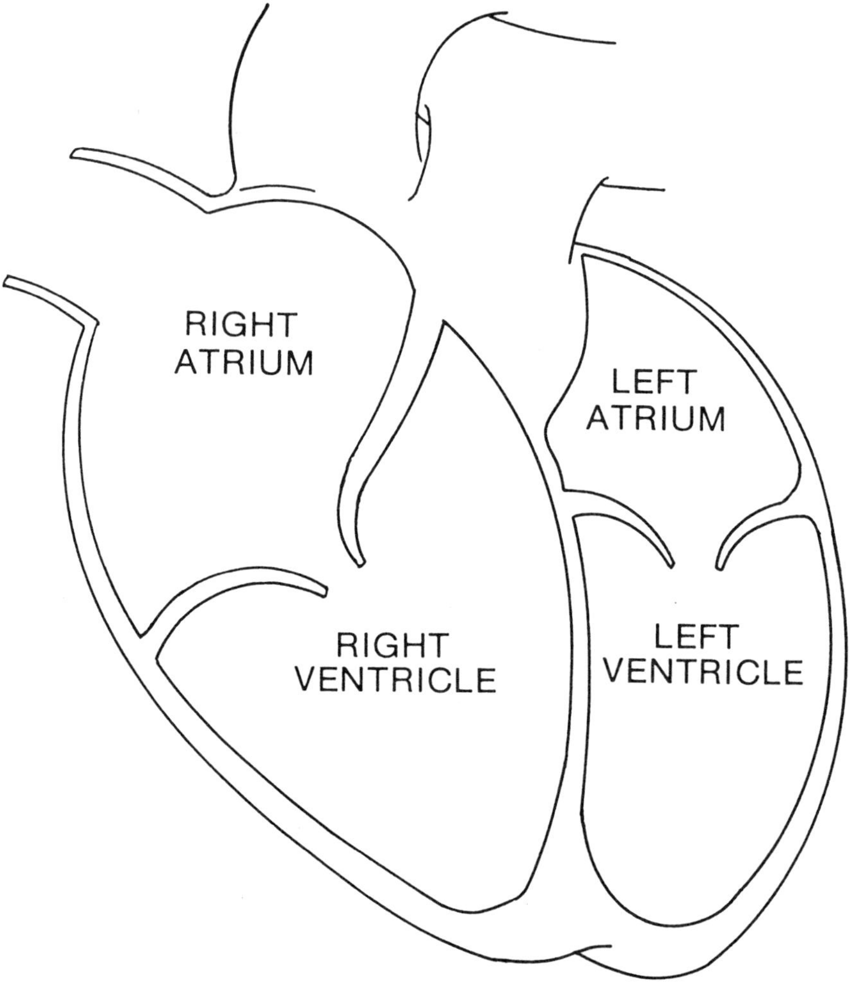

Figure 4.1 The heart is an electro-chemically controlled, double-sided pump that produces a pulsatile blood flow.

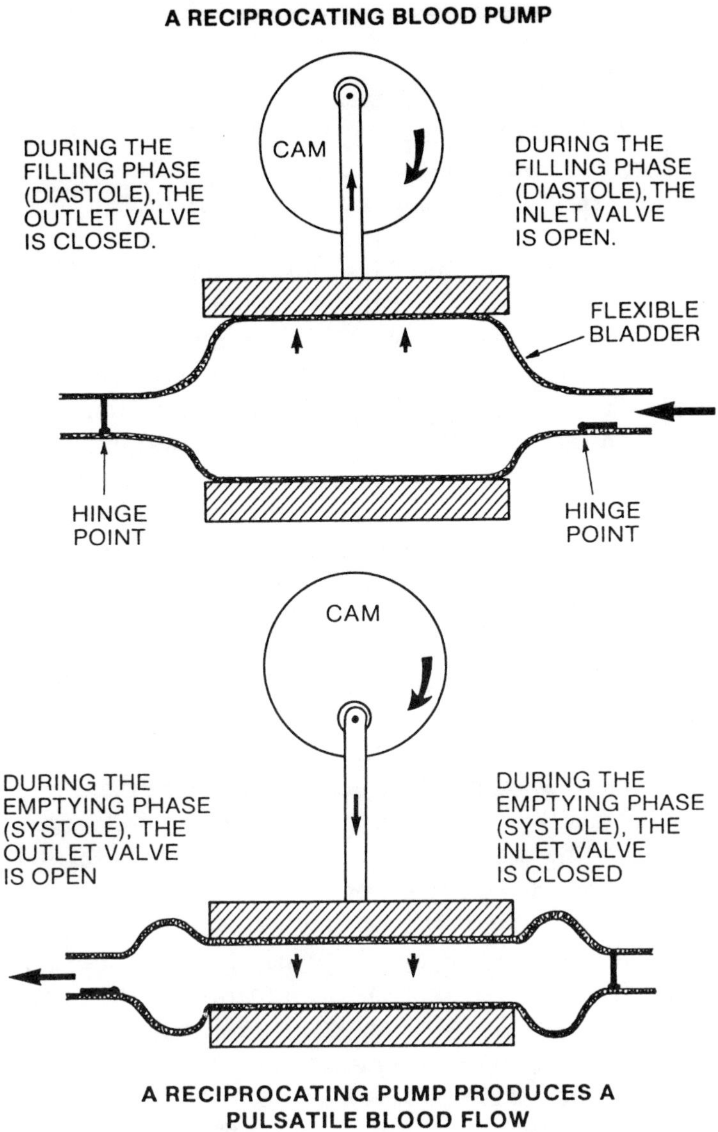

Figure 4.2 A reciprocating pump operates in a manner similar to the human heart.

person to receive a permanent artificial heart implantation.

One kind of rotary pump has been used extensively for open heart surgery—the DeBakey roller-type blood pump (Figure 4.3). Because of its mechanical simplicity and its safety features, most open heart teams rely upon it. It has withstood the test of time. This pump displaces (propels) blood from the inlet to the outlet by a rotating piece and by compressing the tubing against a fixed raceway by rollers. The inside of the tubing can be sterilized easily, while the outside of the tubing can be handled to insert the tubing into the pump head. The roller-type pump can be hand-operated in the event of mechanical or electrical failure. The roller-type pump produces a relatively nonpulsatile blood flow (Figure 4.5). One disadvantage of the roller-type pump is that it creates a very high negative pressure at its inlet side. It is a "sucking pump." It does not fill passively, but rather fills actively—by suction. If not used properly, it can suck in and pump air, creating a very real danger to the patient (Figure 4.6).

Another kind of blood pump, used mostly in the early days of open-heart surgery, was a multiple-finger pump—the sigmamotor pump. As with the roller-type blood pump, the sigmamotor pump "milks" blood from the inlet to the outlet by means of a compressible tube. The outside of the tubing may be handled, while the lumen maintains a sterile pathway. Multiple fingers milk the tube in a peristaltic, wave-like fashion. Sigmamotor pumps are mechanically simple and reliable like the roller-type pumps. However, at high speeds, sigmamotor pumps have been known to produce excessive hemolysis.

Centrifugal-type pumps are becoming increasingly popular in heart-lung circuits (Figure 4.7). Most of these pumps have a rotating impeller (a bladed wheel that "impels" or moves the fluid through the outlet of the pump) which creates a pressure difference between the inlet and outlet sides, causing the fluid to flow in one direction. Centrifugal pumps also produce a nonpulsatile blood flow (Figure 4.8).

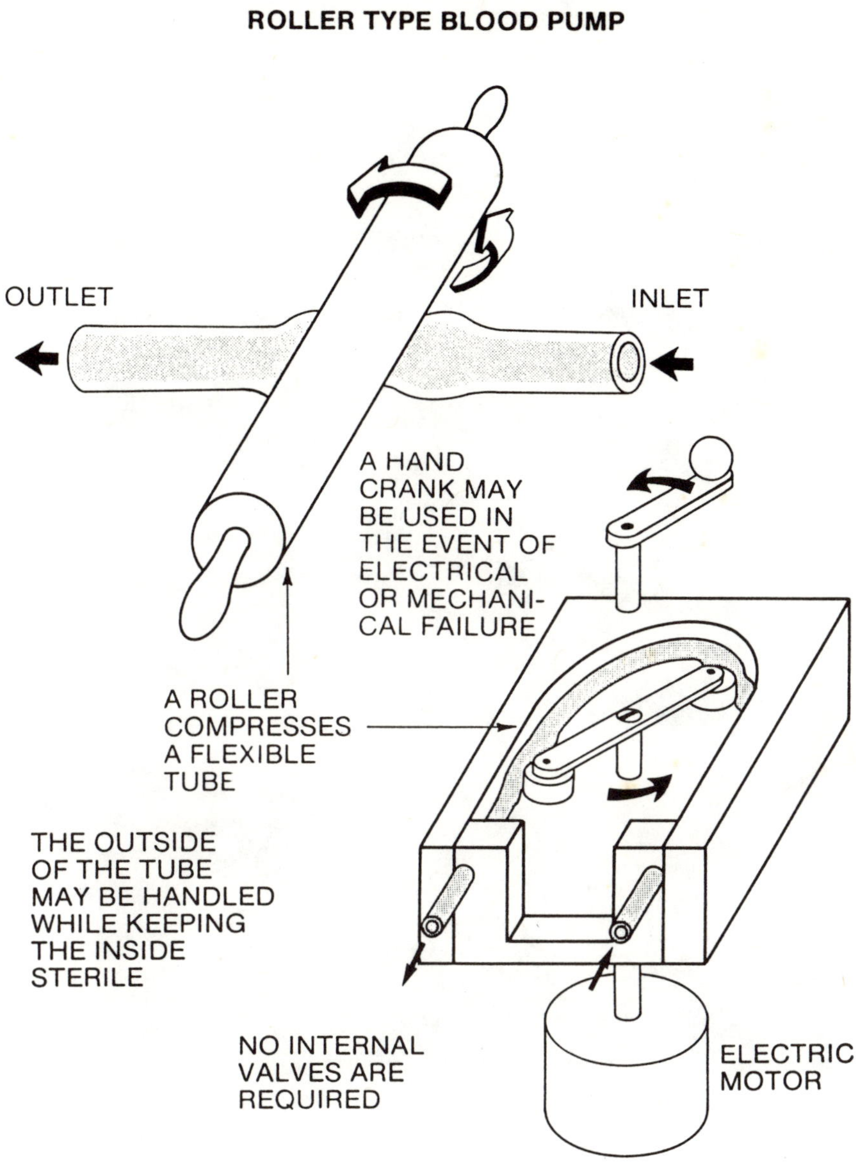

Figure 4.3 The roller-type blood pump is used extensively during heart operations.

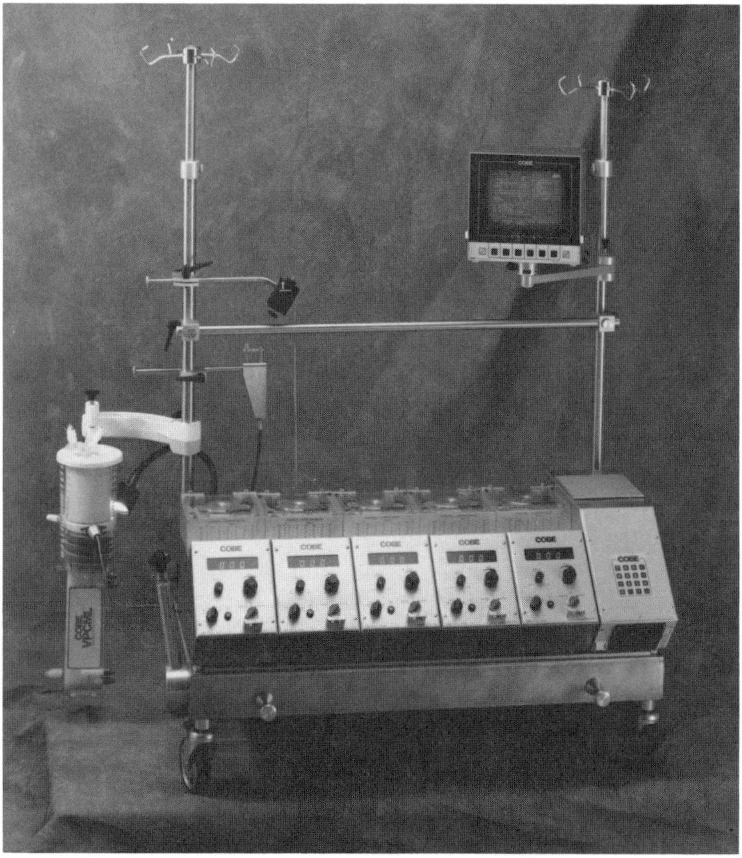

Figure 4.4 Five roller-type blood pumps arepart of this heart-lung machine console. (Courtesy of Cobe Laboratories, Arvada, Colorado.)

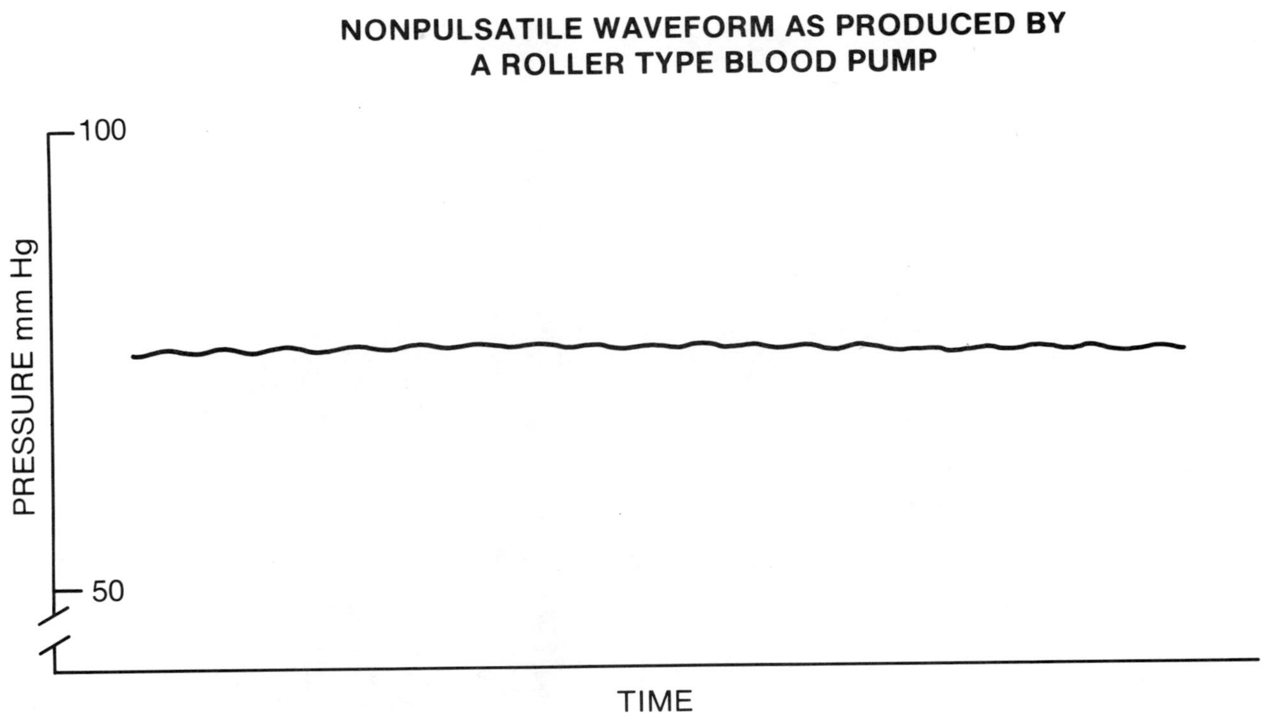

Figure 4.5 A roller-type blood pump produces a relatively non-pulsatile blood flow.

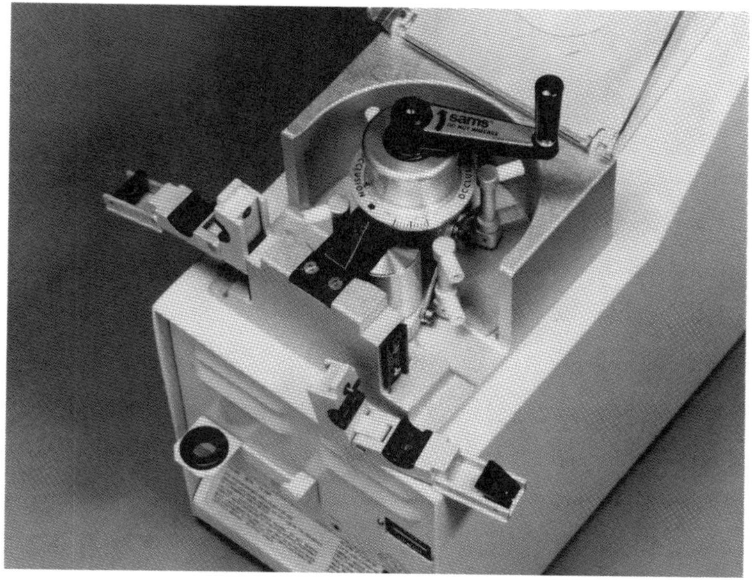

Figure 4.6 A roller-type blood pump with hand crank inserted in case of electrical or mechanical failure. (Courtesy of Sarns, 3M Healthcare, Ann Arbor, Michigan.)

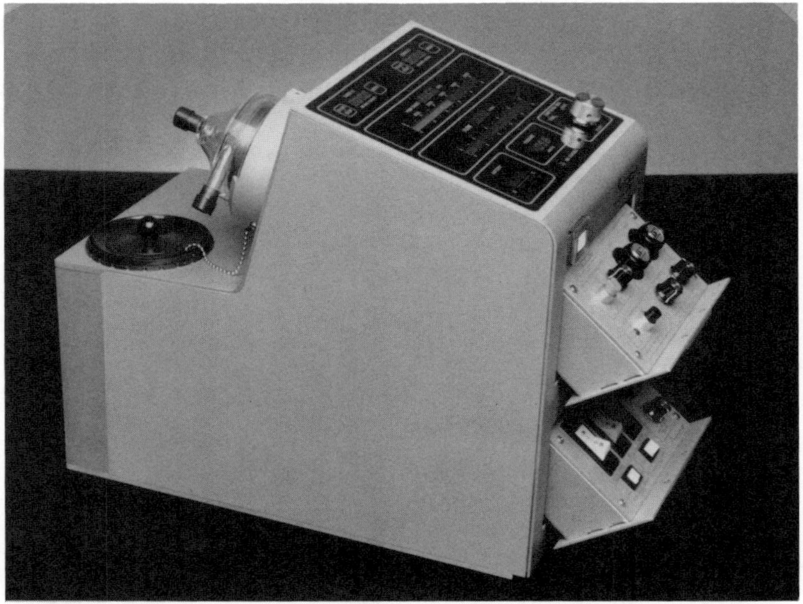

Figure 4.7 A disposable centrifugal-type blood pump. (Courtesy of Biomedicus, Eden Prairie, Minnesota.)

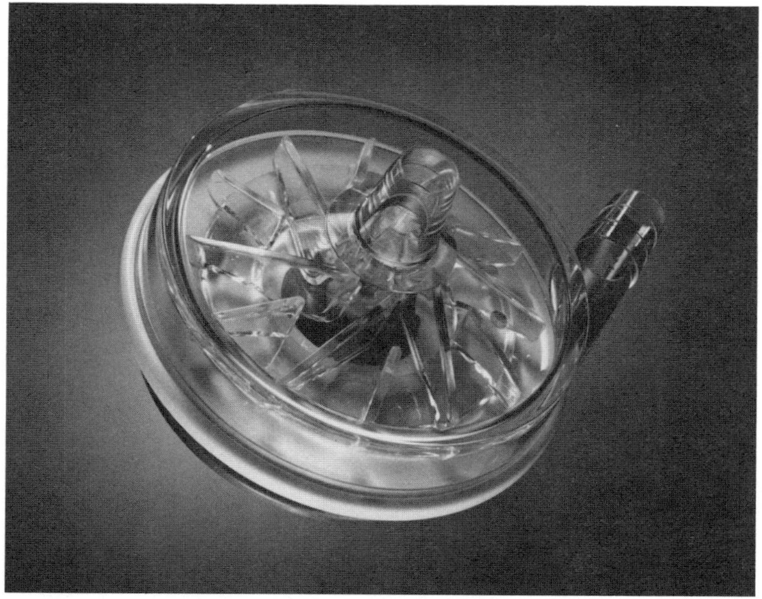

Figure 4.8 A disposable centrigual-type blood pump. (Courtesy of Sarns, 3M Healthcare, Ann Arbor, Michigan.)

Whether or not a pulsatile flow (being more physiologically "normal") is necessary to a blood pump is a controversial point (Figure 4.9). Galletti and Brecher, in their book, *Heart-Lung Bypass*, say, "The pulsatile action appears to be the solution reached by nature for obtaining maximal pumping efficiency by a hollow muscle. There is at present no conclusive evidence that a mechanical system need be likewise." Although *Heart-Lung Bypass* was written in 1962, and although there have been several convincing articles written which propose that pulsatile flow benefits normal physiology, the evidence is still inconclusive. Indeed, some natural circulatory flow *is* continuous—in the capillary beds, for example.

Uses of Pumps in the Extracorporeal Circuit

Several blood pumps are used in the typical extracorporeal circuit. The main, or arterial pump, propels oxygenated blood to the patient's body.

A blood pump may also be used as a left ventricular vent pump. That is, it is used to return blood from the left ventricle by means of a catheter placed either in the superior pulmonary vein or in the apex of the left ventricle. This left ventricular vent blood is pumped from the left ventricle to a cardiotomy reservoir (Figure 4.10). The blood in the cardiotomy reservoir then returns to the extracorporeal circuit following filtration to remove debris. An additional part of the cardiotomy reservoir system is a hand-held cardiotomy suction. This device returns blood from the open heart surgical field or from an open cardiac chamber to the cardiotomy reservoir by means of yet another blood pump. After filtration, this blood is also eventually returned to the extracorporeal circuit (Figure 4.12). The cardiotomy suction system has one important disadvantage. It has been demonstrated to increase the amount of damage to the fragile cellular and noncellular components of the blood. The cardiotomy suction system should be used only when necessary by the surgical team, and used at a low operating speed.

PULSATILE PRESSURE WAVEFORM AS PRODUCED BY THE HEART OR A PULSATILE BLOOD PUMP

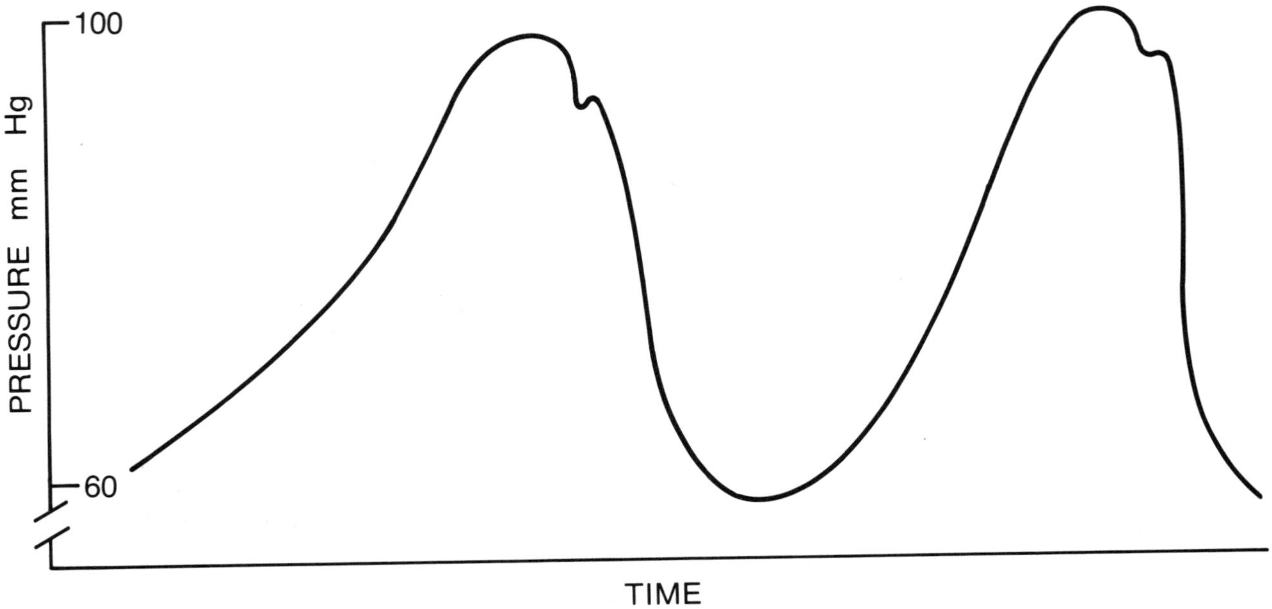

Figure 4.9

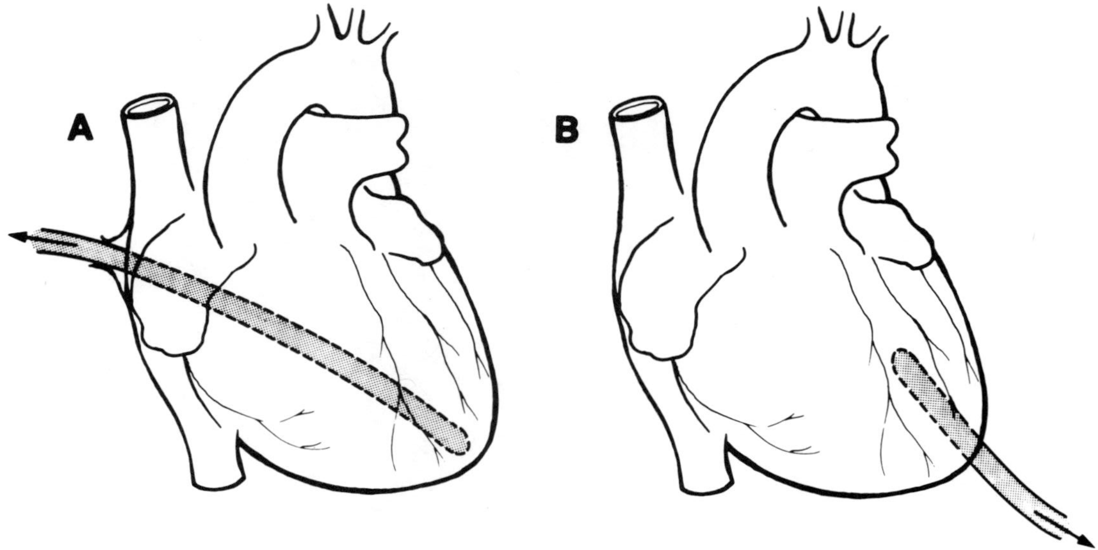

Figure 4.10 (A) The left ventricle may be vented by a catheter inserted through the superior pulmonary vein and advanced through the mitral valve, or (B) by a catheter inserted into the apex of the left ventricle.

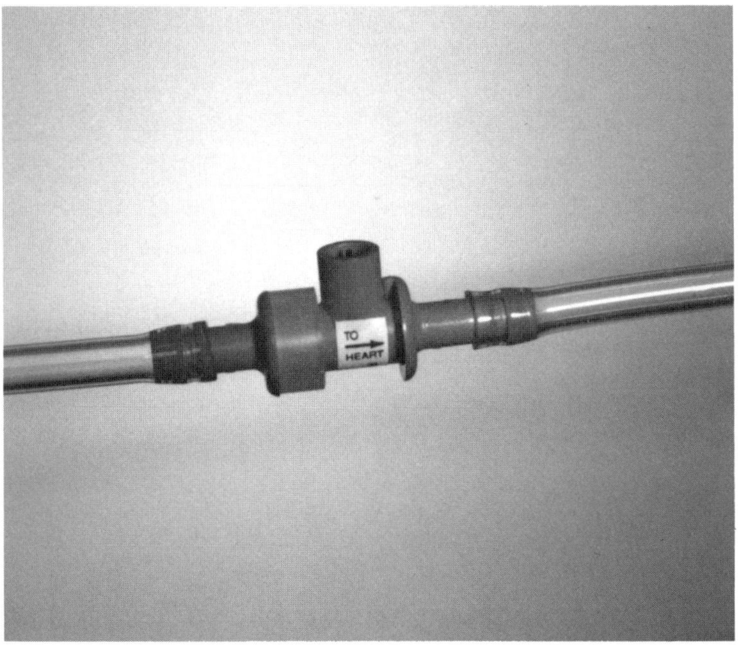

Figure 4.11 This suction control valve relieves suction when the cannula is occluded. It can be used with left ventricular venting. (Courtesy American Omni Medical, Inc., Costa Mesa, California.)

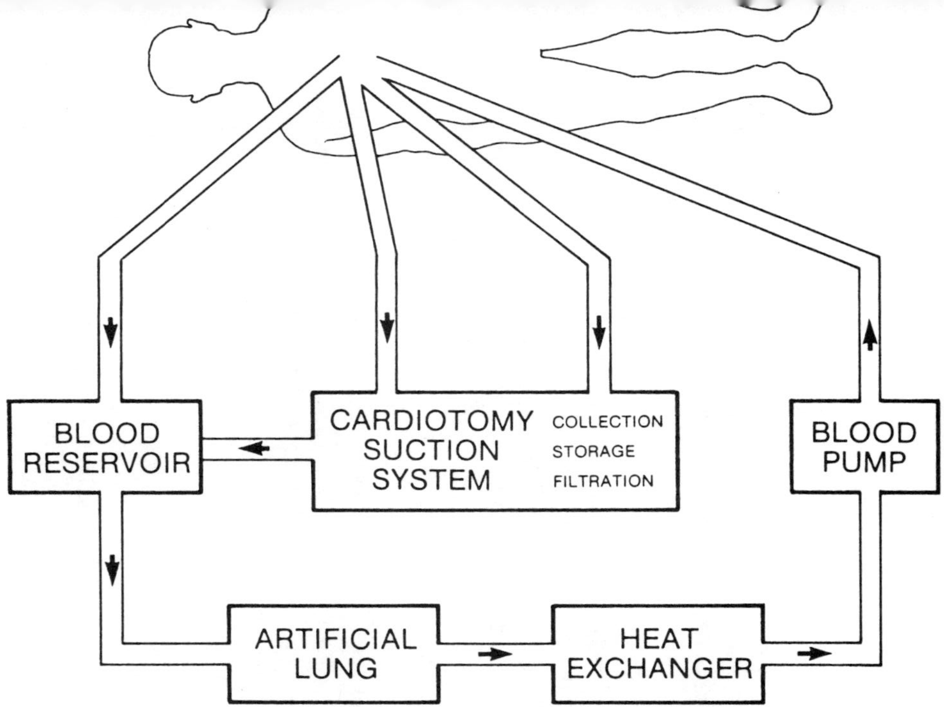

Figure 4.12 The cardiotomy suction system collects, filters, and stores the blood.

LUNGS & OTHER GAS EXCHANGE DEVICES

CHAPTER FIVE

The Natural Lung

The function of the natural lungs is to add oxygen and to remove carbon dioxide from the blood. This function occurs while the blood passes through the alveolar capillary network (Figure 5.1).

Deoxygenated blood from the body's venous system returns to the right atrium and is pumped on to the right ventricle. The right ventricle pumps the deoxygenated blood through the pulmonary valve into the pulmonary artery to reach the lungs and the pulmonary capillary network. Oxygenation then takes place and the oxygenated blood is returned through the four pulmonary veins to the left atrium. The left atrium moves the blood through the mitral valve into the left ventricle. The left ventricle contracts, forcing the oxygenated blood out through the aortic valve and out into the systemic circulation. Once in the systemic circulation, oxygenated blood passes through increasingly smaller vessels—from arteries, to arterioles, to capillaries. In the capillary beds, the blood transfers its oxygen to the cells and takes on carbon dioxide and other wastes. The deoxygenated blood goes through a reverse process and eventually reaches the right heart once more.

Alveolus

The process of gas exchange in the alveolar-capillary level of the lungs takes place by diffusion (Figure 5.2). Gases diffuse from a region of higher concentration (pressure) to a region of lower concentration (pressure). Diffusion of a gas can be illustrated by the action of a organic chemical compound known as "mercaptan." In its gaseous form, one part is mixed with 20,000,000 parts of natural gas. It is the

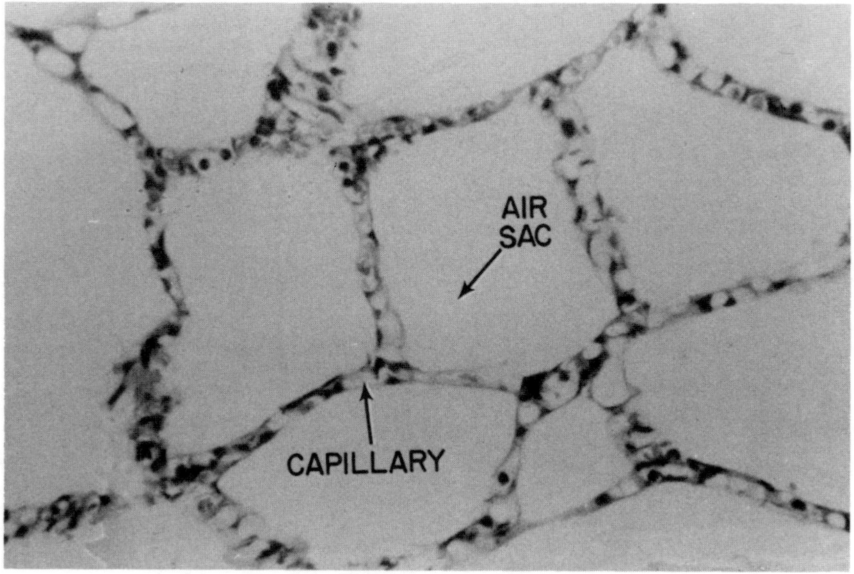

Figure 5.1 An alveolus (air sac) is seen along with its pulmonary capillary. (Courtesy of St. Luke's Medical Center, Pathology Department, Phoenix, Arizona.)

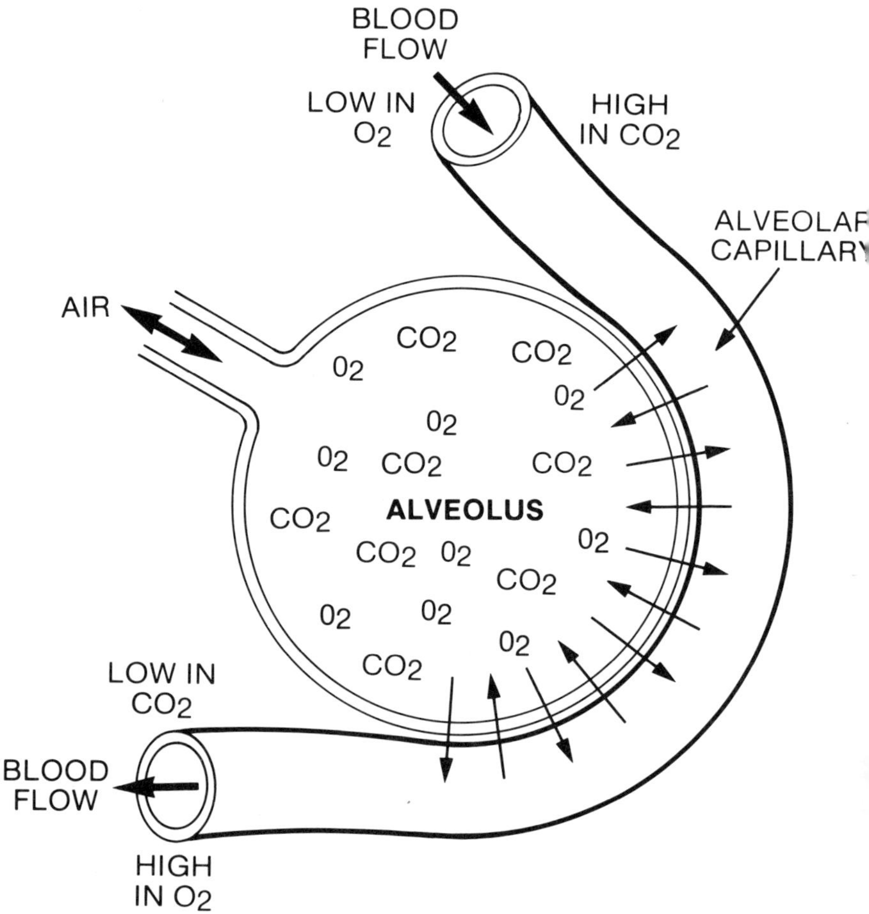

Figure 5.2 Diffusion across the alveolar (pulmonary) membrane.

diffusion of mercaptan that gives natural gas its distinctive bad (sulphuric) odor.

The composition and concentration of gases found in the alveoli are determined by (1) the composition and concentration of the air we breathe, and (2) by the mechanical process of ventilation—moving air in and out of the lungs. Fresh air is composed of approximately 79% nitrogen, 20.96% oxygen, and .04% carbon dioxide. Additional quantities of water vapor and other gases are also present.

These gases follow natural laws. For example, Dalton's Law states that the total pressure exerted by all gases found in a given environment is equal to the sum of the pressures of each individual gas. Each gas, it can be said, exerts a "partial pressure" of the total pressure exerted by all gases in that environment. Partial pressure is denoted in scientific writing by the upper case letter "P" that precedes the gas's chemical symbol, for example, PO_2, PCO_2, PN_2, etc. Thus, according to Dalton's Law, the barometric pressure of atmospheric air equals the sum of the pressures of the gases present in the atmosphere: $BP = PO_2 + PCO_2 + PN_2 + PH_2O$. The average barometric pressure of air at sea level is 760 millimeters of mercury. Water vapor exerts a partial pressure of 47 millimeters of mercury at normal body temperature (37° C). If barometric pressure were measured at 760 millimeters of mercury *minus* 47 millimeters of mercury (the partial pressure of water vapor), we can deduce that dry barometric pressure would equal 713 millimeters of mercury. An example of calculated partial pressures of N_2, O_2, and CO_2, based on percentage, is illustrated in Figure 5.3.

Artificial Lungs

Artificial lungs perform exactly the same function as natural lungs. The terms "oxygenator" and "artificial lung" are used interchangeably by the medical profession. "Artificial lung" is perhaps the more accurate term since the artificial lung not only oxygenates the blood, but is also responsible for removing carbon dioxide from the blood. The artificial lung must remove carbon dioxide in the correct

PARTIAL PRESSURE OF GASES

GAS	% CONCENTRATION		ATMOSPHERIC PRESSURE (DRY)		PARTIAL PRESSURE
NITROGEN	0.79	X	713	=	563.3
OXYGEN	0.2096	X	713	=	149.4
CARBON DIOXIDE	0.0004	X	713	=	0.3
	1.0000				713.0

Figure 5.3

proportions to avoid excessive accumulation of carbon dioxide (causing respiratory acidosis) or to avoid eliminating too much carbon dioxide (causing respiratory alkalosis).

Artificial lungs have been divided into three general categories: the bubble-type artificial lung, the membrane-type artificial lung, and the film-type artificial lung. We will discuss them in order (Figure 5.4).

Bubble-type Artificial Lungs:

The basis for the use of the "bubble oxygenator" is the fact that oxygen can be dispersed directly into the blood, and, as a result, gas exchange will take place across the blood-gas interface. The amount of gas exchanged by the bubble is in direct proportion to the total surface area created by the bubbles. To increase the amount of gas transfer (O_2 or O_2 + CO_2), one simply increases the gas flow rate. Carbon dioxide is eliminated from the oxygenated blood by being carried upward in the bubble to be dispersed to the atmosphere. Most bubble-type oxygenators require that carbon dioxide be mixed with the oxygen to prevent the elimination of too much carbon dioxide.

Bubble-type oxygenators are composed of two separate compartments or chambers (Figures 5.5, 5.6, and 5.7). The first chamber contains the bubble or oxygenator column in which bubbles of gas are dispersed into the venous blood that flows into the chamber. Gas exchange takes place by direct blood-gas interface (Figure 5.8). This oxygenated blood then flows over a baffle into an arterial reservoir, sometimes referred to as a "de-bubbling" or a "de-foaming" reservoir. After this de-bubbling process, the oxygenated blood is returned to the patient's body.

It is very important that gas flow to bubble oxygenators be carefully regulated. First, excessive gas flows can damage the fragile, formed elements of the blood by the "jetting" effect of the gas as it flows rapidly into the blood. This trauma to the blood is a time-related phenomenon—the longer a patient is on cardiopulmonary bypass, the more blood trauma one might expect to see. Second, an excessive amount of gas flow to the bubble oxygenator creates an

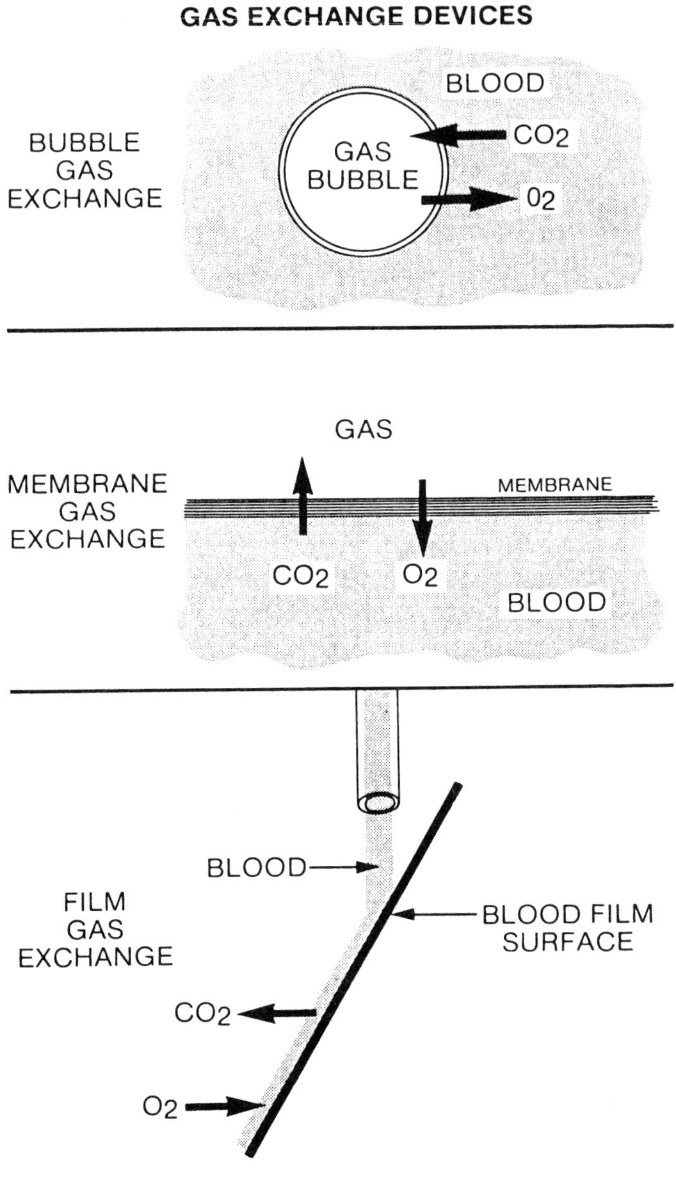

Figure 5.4 Three general categories of artificial lungs are the bubble-type, the membrane-type, and the film-type.

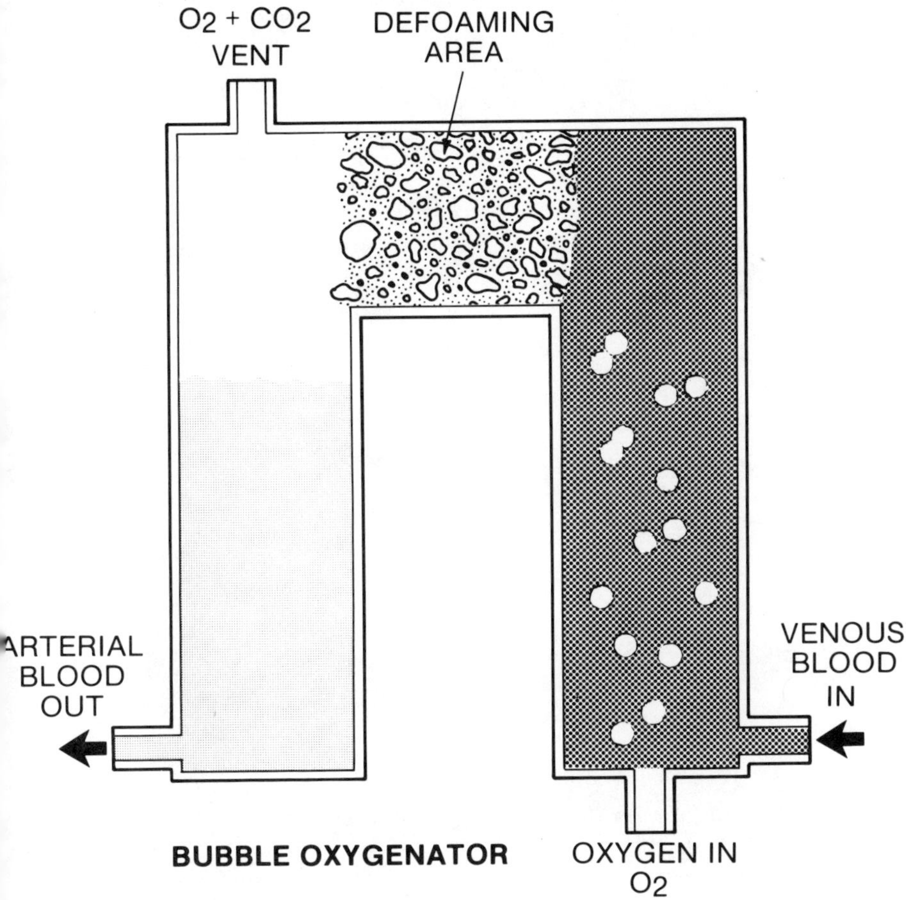

Figure 5.5 The bubble-type oxygenator exposes blood to a direct blood-gas interface.

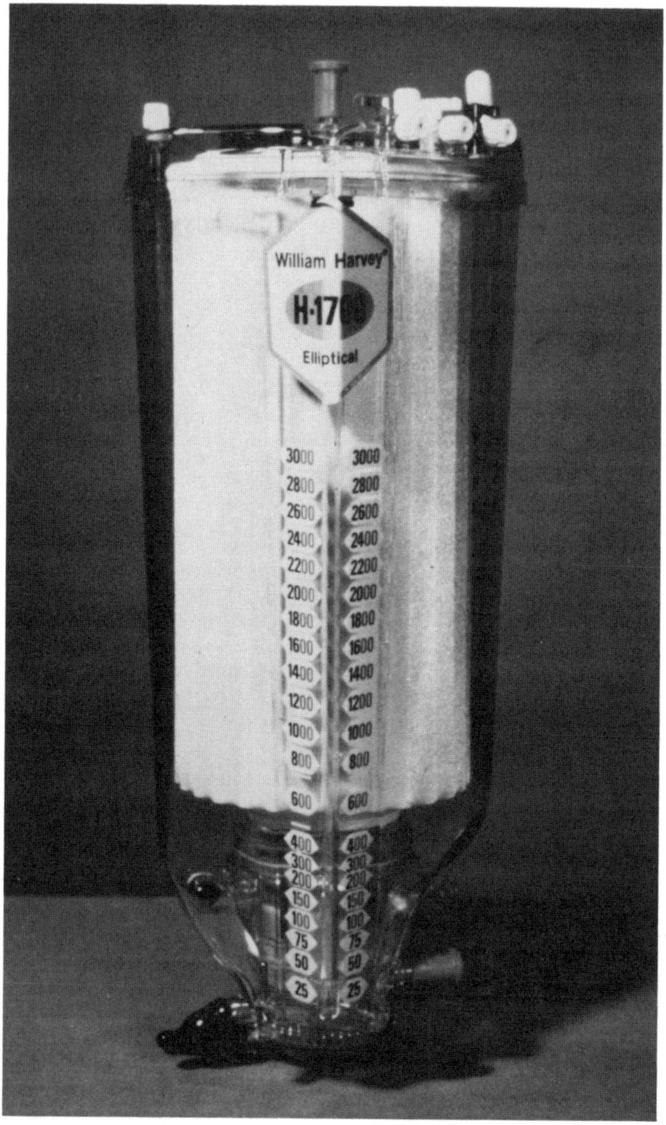

Figure 5.6 A modern bubble-type oxygenator. (Courtesy of Bard Cardiopulmonary Division, C.R. Bard, Inc., Billerica, Massachuetts.)

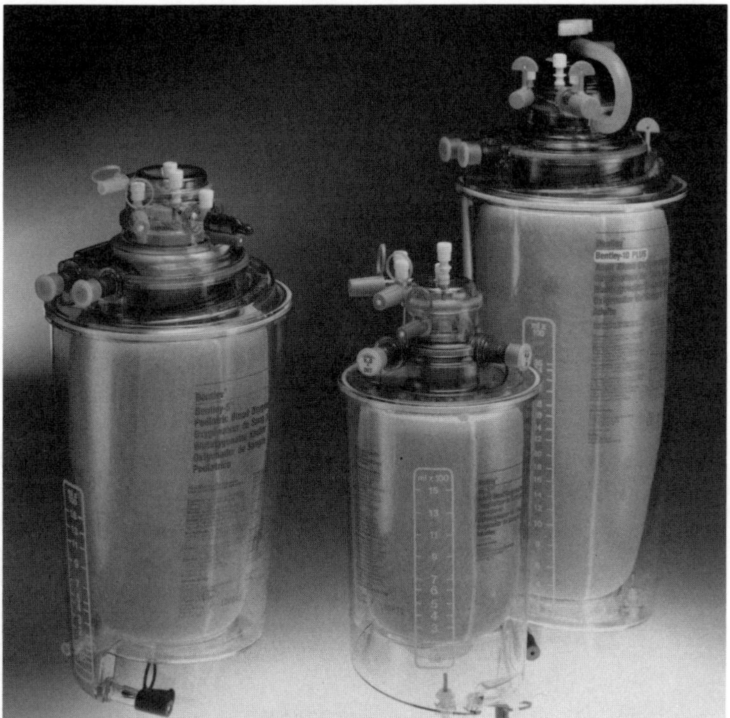

Figure 5.7 Pediatric, infant, and adult models of bubble oxygenators. (Courtesy of Baxter Healthcare Corporation, Bentley Laboratories Division, Irvine, California.)

excessive number of gas bubbles that are difficult to eliminate. Any of the bubbles that escape into the arterial bloodstream can result in harmful emboli, and the smaller the bubbles, the more difficult they are to remove. To help remove bubbles, the de-bubbling chambers of bubble oxygenators are equipped with plastic sponges which have been coated with a silicone compound. This silicone preparation decreases the surface tension of the bubbles, causing them to burst. Secondarily, the foam sponges act as gross filters for any debris which might accumulate in this chamber.

Membrane-type Artificial Lungs:

Unlike the bubble oxygenator, the membrane-type artificial lung does not have a direct blood-gas interface. Instead, it has a permeable membrane between the blood side and the gas side of the membrane through which gas exchange takes place by diffusion (Figure 5.8).

The membranes used in membrane-type oxygenators are artificial. Some of the more popular materials used today are: polypropolene, silicone rubber, and expanded polytetrafluroethylene (Teflon) (Figure 5.10).

There are three commonly-used membrane oxygenators. One type is a flat plate membrane oxygenator with the plates folded accordion-style (Figures 5.11 and 5.12. Blood flows on one side of the plates, and gas flows on the opposite side. A second type is a capillary membrane oxygenator in which the blood flows on the inside of the capillaries (each of which is about 200 microns in diameter), and the gas flows on the outside of the capillaries (Figures 5.13 and 5.14). The third type is designed so that gas flows through the capillaries and blood flows around the capillaries. The accordion folds and the multiple capillaries are both attempts to increase the total surface area of the membrane. Total gas transfer is dependent upon the total surface area of the membrane in which gas exchange can take place (Figure 5.15).

Gas exchange takes place by diffusion across a permeable membrane just as it occurs in the natural lung.

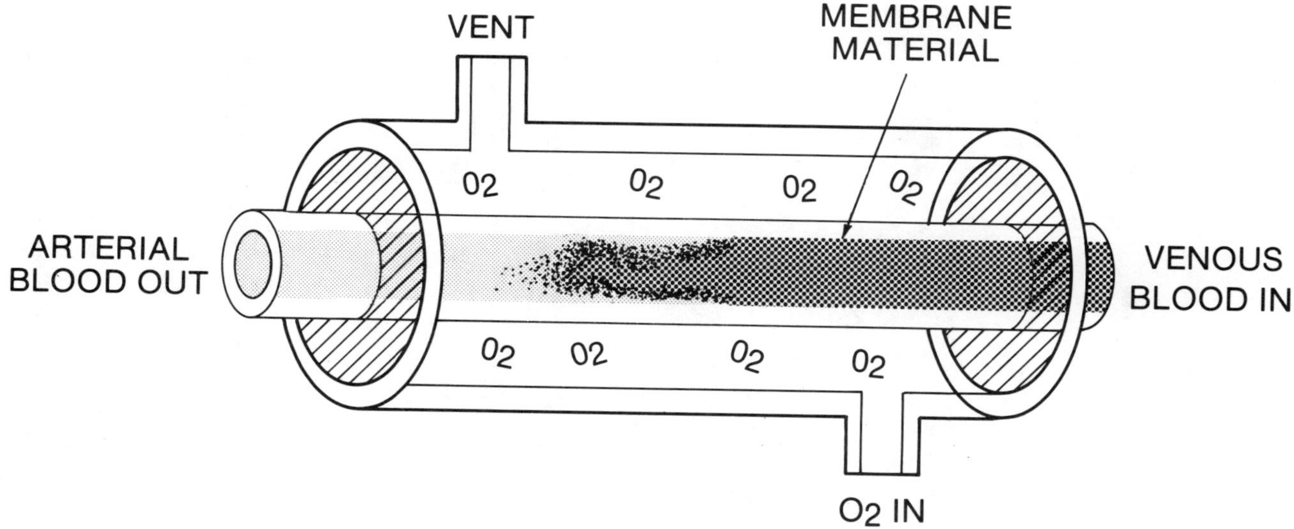

Figure 5.8 Gas exchange takes place in a membrane-type artificial lung through a permeable gas membrane.

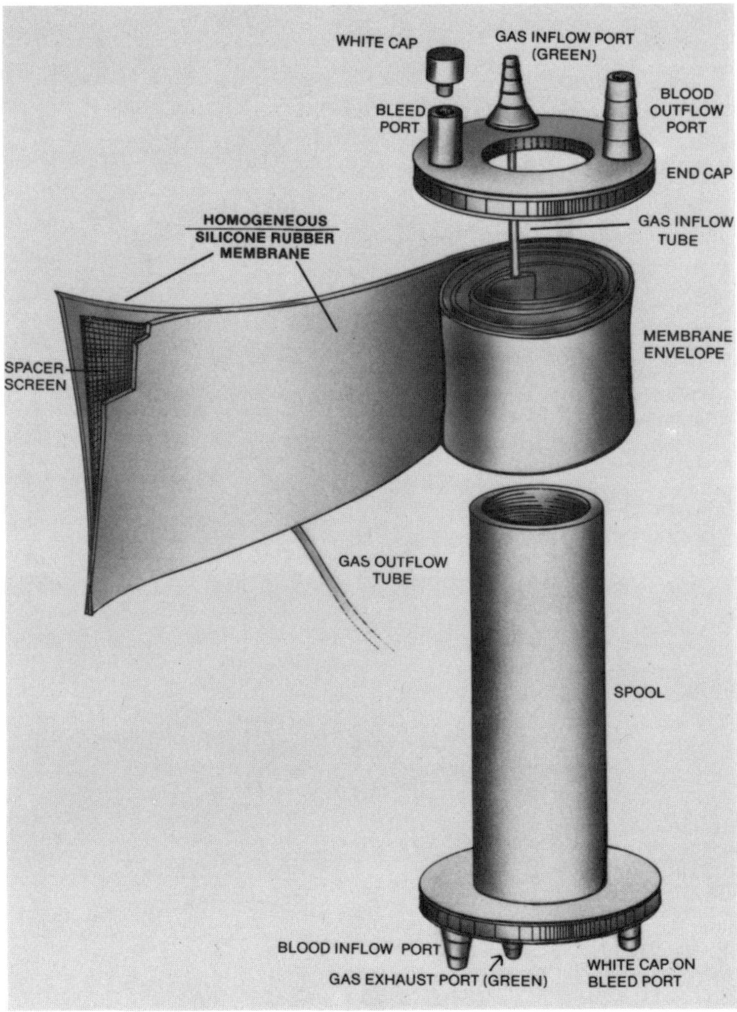

Figure 5.9 Basic assembly configuration of a spiral-wound silicone membrance oxygenator. (Courtesy of SCIMED Life Systems, Inc., Minneapolis, Minnesota.)

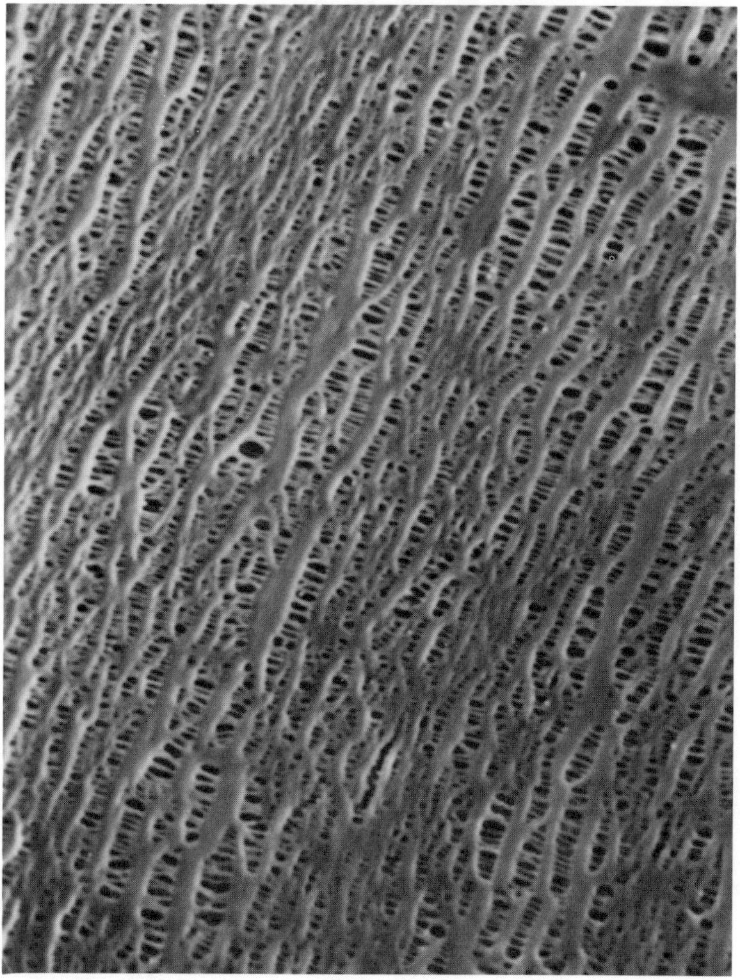

Figure 5.10 A microphotograph (magnified approximately 8,000X) of a polypropene membrane. (Courtesy of the Terumo Company, Piscataway,New Jersey.)

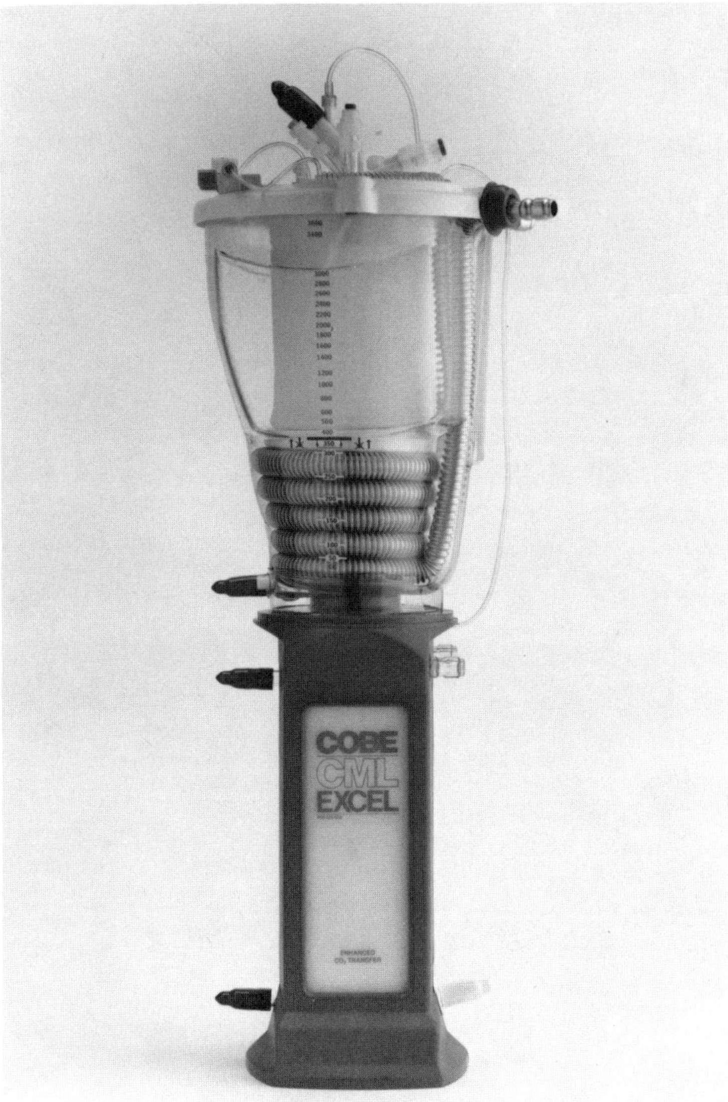

Figure 5.11 An example of a membrane oxygenation system. (Courtesy of Cobe Laboratories, Aravada, Colorado.)

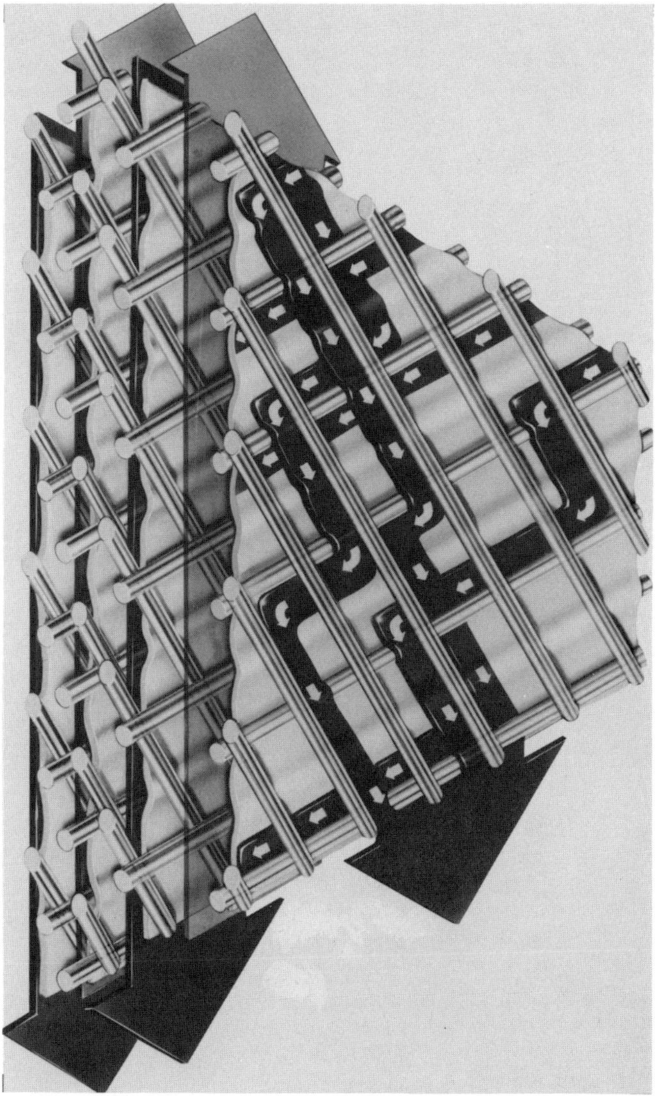

Figure 5.12 The blood flows across baffles or channels in order to increase gas exchange in this membrane oxygenator. (Courtesy of Shiley Laboratories, Santa Ana, California.)

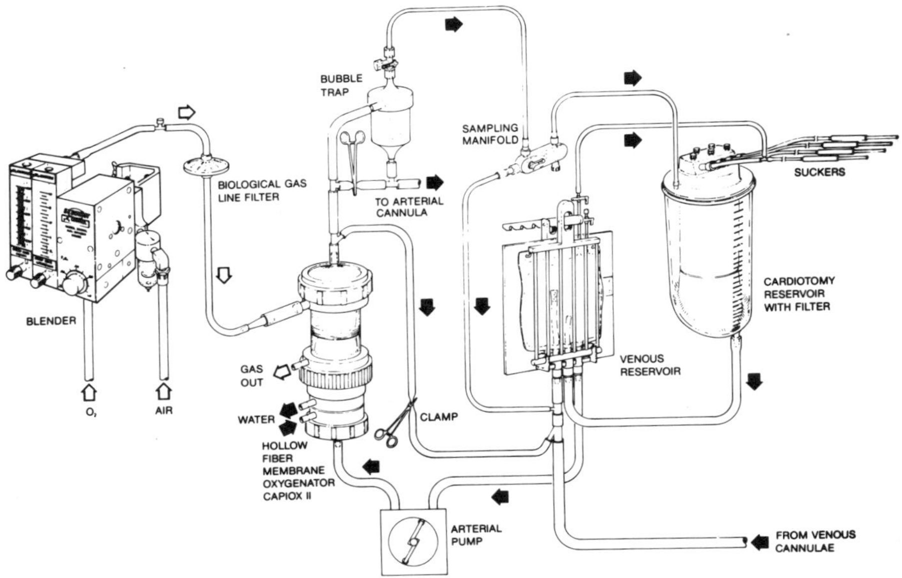

Figure 5.13 A schematic diagram of a membrane oxygenation system complete with cardiotomy reservoir, venous reservoir, inline arterial filter, and gas blender. (Courtesy of the Terumo Company, Piscataway, New Jersey.)

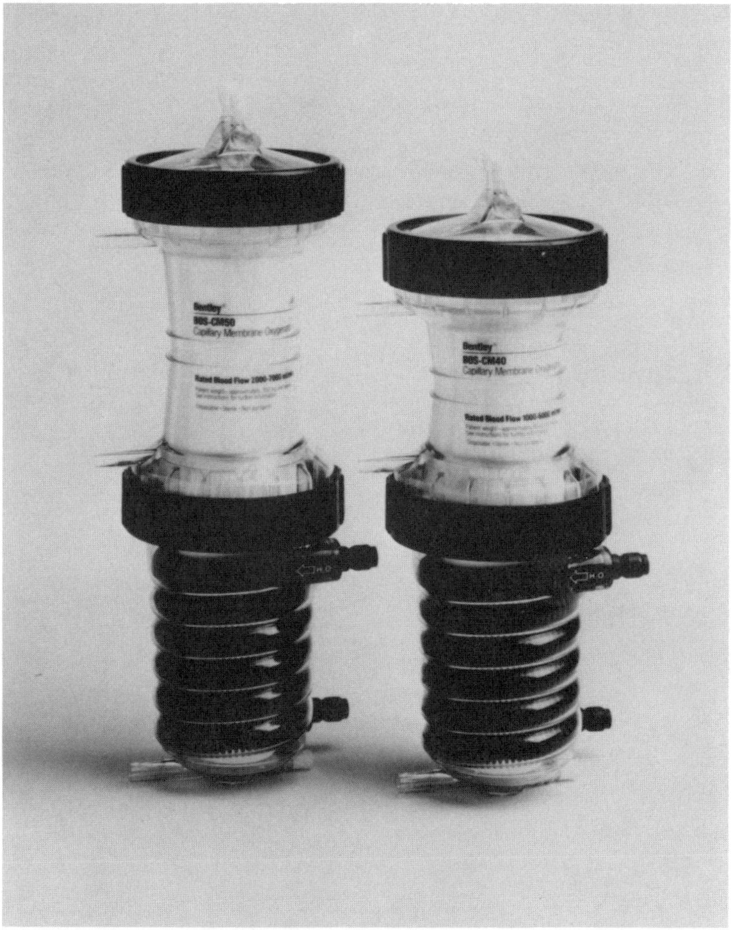

Figure 5.14 Various sizes of membrane oxygenators are used to accomplish both adult and pediatric perfusion. (Courtesy of Baxter Healthcare Corporation, Bentley Laboratories Division, Irvine, California.)

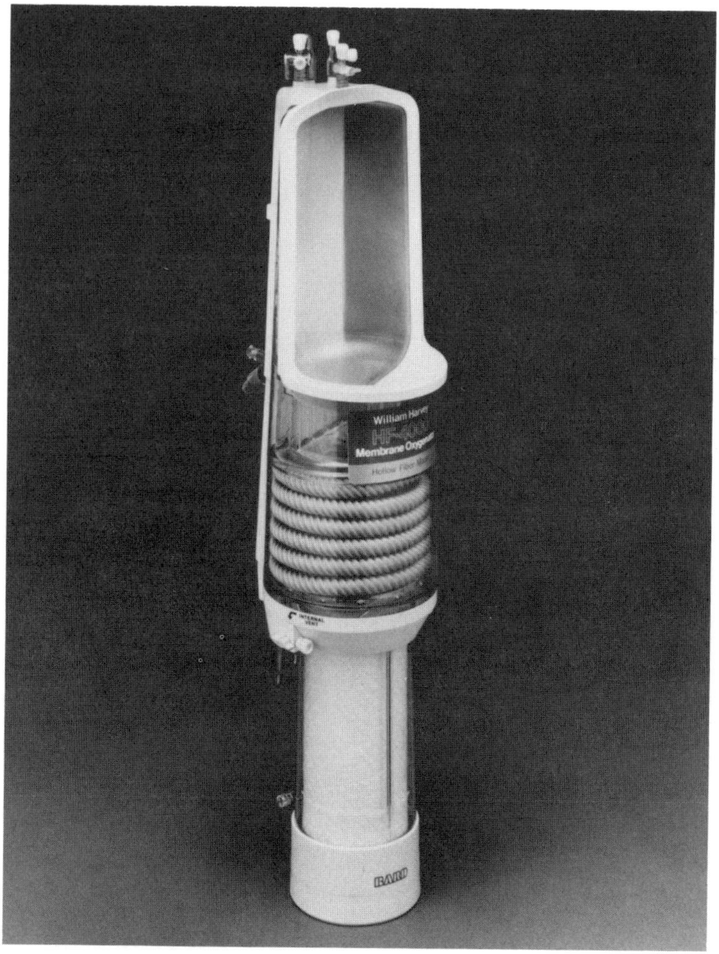

Figure 5.15 This membrane oxygenator has a built-in, collapsible blood reservoir. (Courtesy of Bard Cardiosurgery Division, Billerica, Massachusetts.)

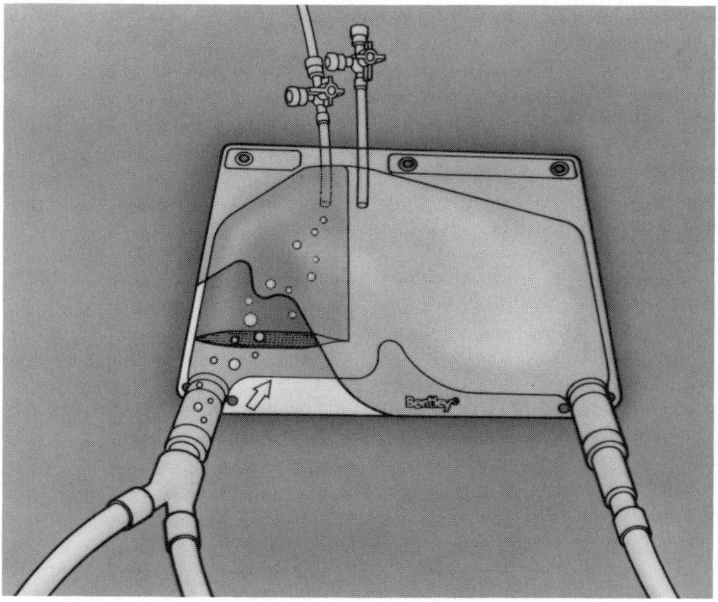

Figure 5.16 A closed venous reservoir that provides for separation and elimination of air coming from the venous line. (Courtesy of Baxter Healthcare Corporation, Bentley Laboratories Division, Irvine, California.)

One may vary the partial pressure on the gas side of the membrane in order to obtain varying partial pressures of gases on the blood side of the membrane. Carbon dioxide may be eliminated more rapidly in a membrane oxygenator by increasing the oxygen flow rate, causing the gas to flow or "sweep" more rapidly across the membrane surface area.

Membrane oxygenators have the reputation of superior blood-handling qualities compared with other oxygenation systems.

Disadvantages generally associated with membrane oxygenators are that they are more expensive than other types, and that they are more complex to use.

Film-type Artificial Lungs:
Many of the early gas exchange devices were of the film-type (Figure 5.17). We mention them here, mostly because of their historical interest. Venous blood was spread in a thin film over a screen or baffle, exposed to an oxygen-rich atmosphere, then collected in an arterial reservoir for perfusion to the patient. Although these devices worked adequately as oxygenators, they had several major disadvantages—they required a large priming volume, they were difficult to clean and sterilize, and their assembly required a great degree of attention to detail (Figure 5.21).

Experimental Variations

There are some interesting experimental variations of the three basic types of artificial lungs. For example, the liquid-liquid interface artificial lungs use the principle that blood will not mix with certain liquids. As a result, liquid fluorocarbons and liquid silicones have been used. These fluids can carry large amounts of oxygen and carbon dioxide in solution. The fluids are saturated with oxygen. Then a flow of the saturated fluid is apposed to a flow of blood. At the point of apposition, gas exchange takes place. Then, in another process, separation of the transfer fluid and the blood takes place. Some of these liquid-liquid systems, although complicated, have been reported to have excellent blood-handling characteristics. However, a major problem

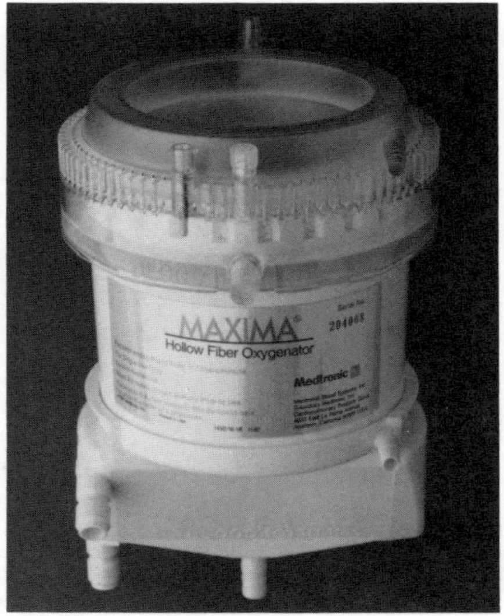

Figure 5.17 An example of a membrane-type, capillary artificial lung in which the gas flows on the inside of the capillary and the blood flows on the outside of the capillary. (Courtesy Medtronic Blood Systems, Inc., Anaheim, California.)

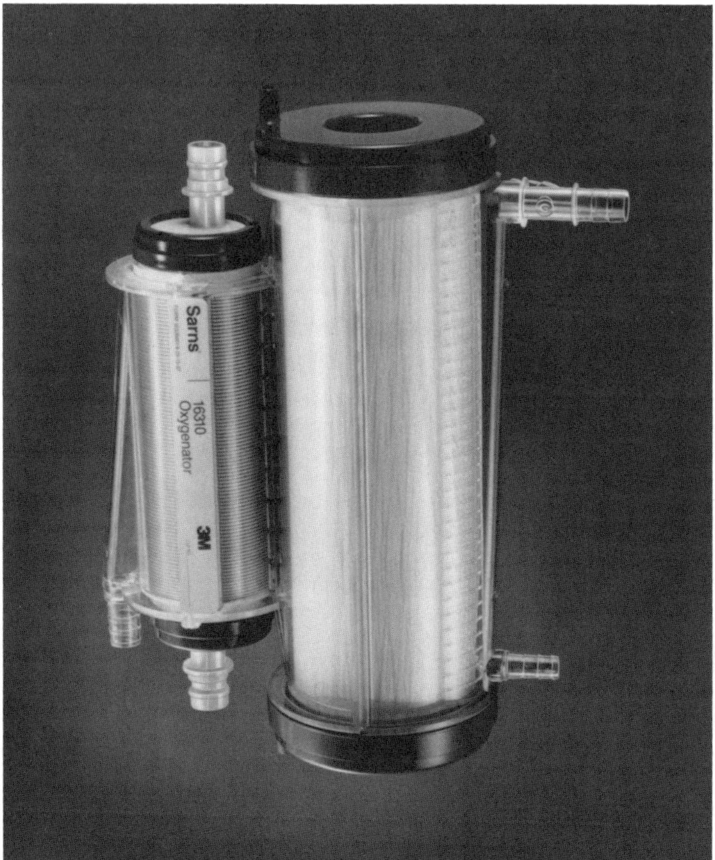

Figure 5.18 Another example of a membrane oxygenator with an integral heat exchanger. (Courtesy of Sarns, 3M Healthcare, Ann Arbor, Michigan.)

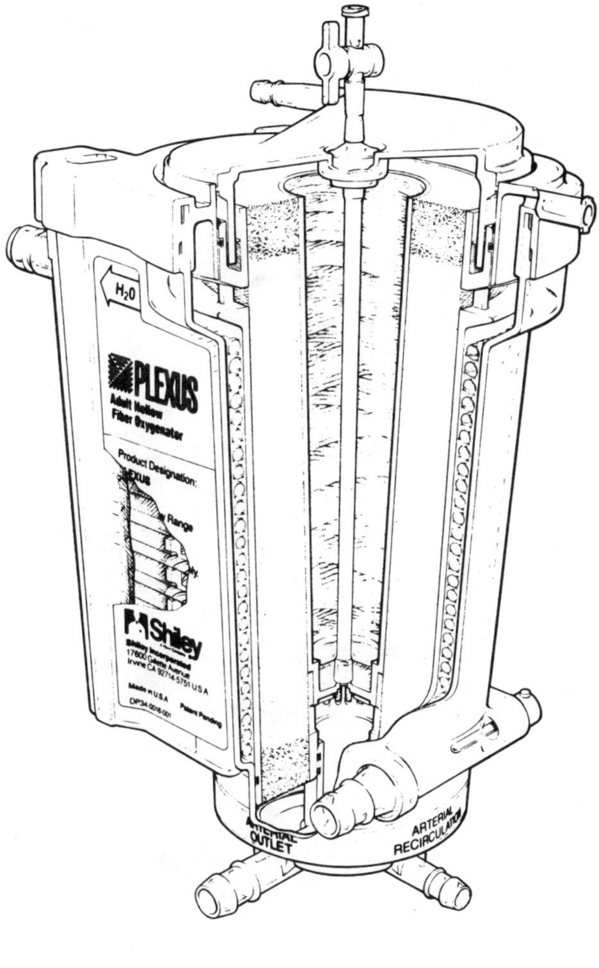

Figure 5.19 This membrane oxygenator incorporates a venous bubble trap at the top of the unit. Blood enters at the bottom, flows up through the heat exchanger into the bubble trap where air may be purged. (Courtesy of Shiley, Inc., Irvine, California.)

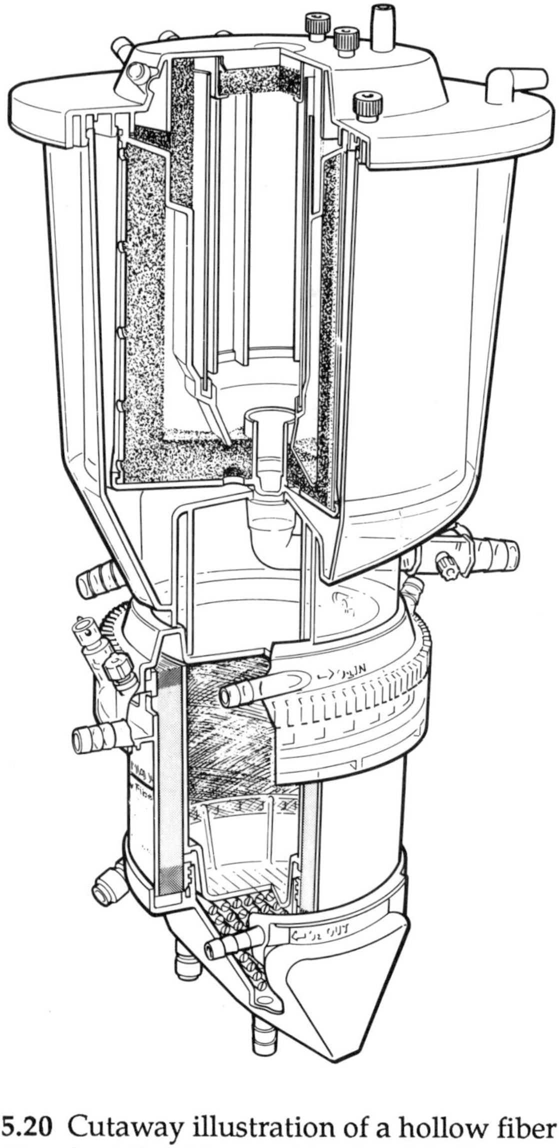

Figure 5.20 Cutaway illustration of a hollow fiber (capillary) artificial lung with a hardshell venous reservoir. (Courtesy of Medtronic Blood Systems, Inc., Anaheim, California.)

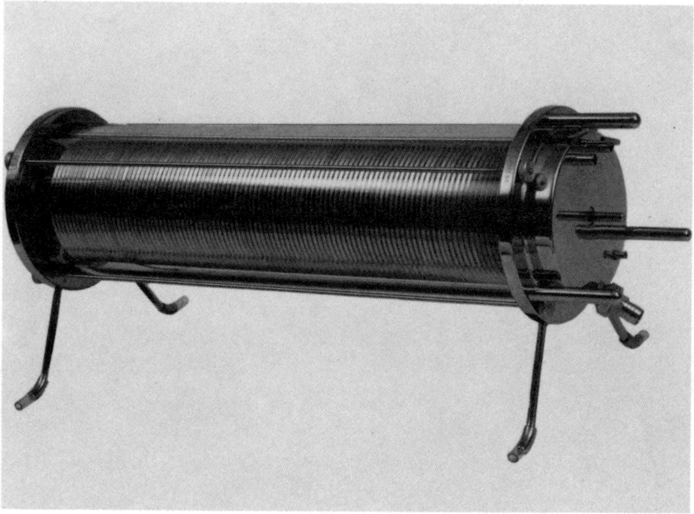

Figure 5.21 A film-type, rotating disc artificial lung. (Courtesy of Sarns Company, 3M Healthcare, Ann Arbor, Michigan.)

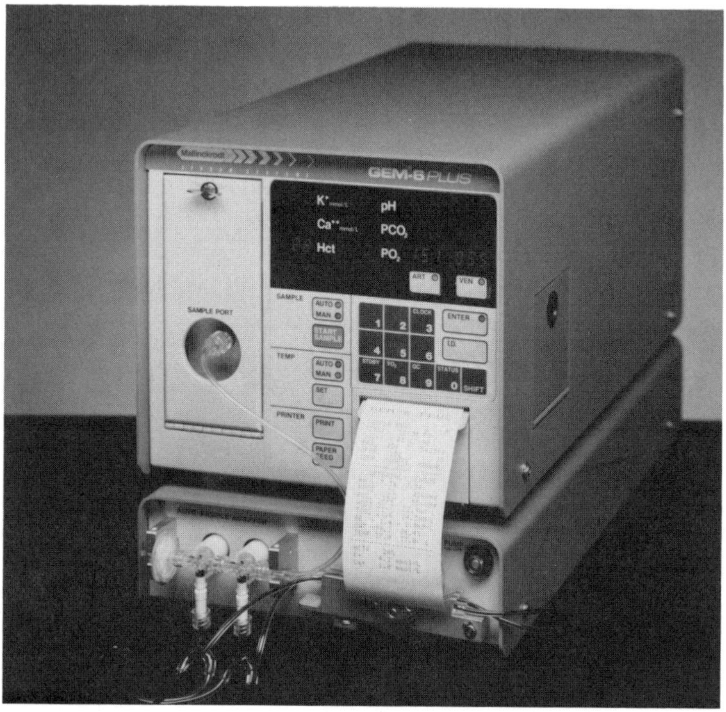

Figure 5.22 This automated blood gas and blood chemistry system is designed for use in cardiovascular surgery. It measures PO_2, PCO_2, pH, Ca^{++}, K^+, and Hct. Blood gases are especially important when evaluating the performance of an oxygenator during open heart surgery. (Courtesy of Mallinckrodt Sensor Systems, Ann Arbor, Michigan.)

with these devices lies in the separation process. The blood and the liquid transfer medium (usually liquid fluorocarbon) must be completely separated, with no residual fluorocarbon. This result has been difficult to achieve. Residual fluorocarbon has unknown long-term effects.

OTHER COMPONENTS OF THE SYSTEM

CHAPTER SIX

Filters

There are two basic types of filters in the extracorporeal circuit: the depth-type filter and the screen-type filter (Figure 6.1). Some filtering systems are composites of the two types. For example, the filters found in cardiotomy reservoirs are usually composite filters (Figure 6.2). Filters are used in arterial lines, in cardiotomy reservoirs, and in bubble-type oxygenation systems.

The principle of the depth-type filter is that fibrous material is loosely packed in a container, and filtration takes place by adhesion of debris particles onto the fibers. The screen-type filter, on the other hand, is composed of either wire or fabric mesh. The mesh openings allow for the passage of blood cells of a certain size but entrap larger particles.

One of the problems with filtration systems in the extracorporeal circuit has been how to determine the size of particles that are to be removed (Figure 6.4). As we have seen earlier, blood cells themselves have widely varying diameters—from the platelets, which measure from 2-4 microns; to the leukocytes, which measure from 10-12 microns. Another related problem is based on the fact that blood, as we have mentioned earlier, is not a true liquid but is rather a liquid containing solid suspensions—namely, its formed elements. As a result, it is difficult to remove undesirable elements of the blood, such as dead cells and clumps of cells, without removing some of the desirable elements. For example, when a red cell dies (normally, its life cycle is about 120 days), or when it is overcome by mechanical stresses encountered in an extracorporeal circuit, its cell membrane ruptures and becomes debris that should be removed from the bloodstream. In normal circulation, removal is accomplished by

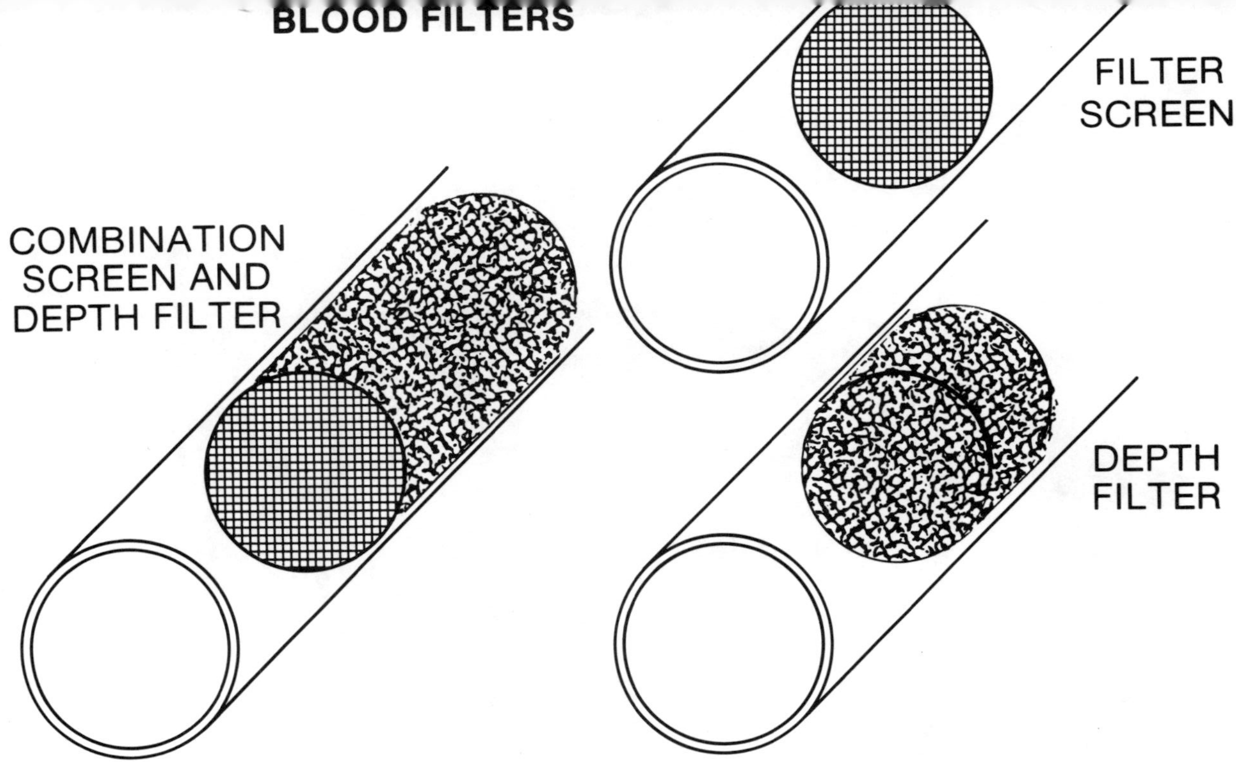

Figure 6.1 Blood filters may be classified as depth-type, screen-type, or a combination of both.

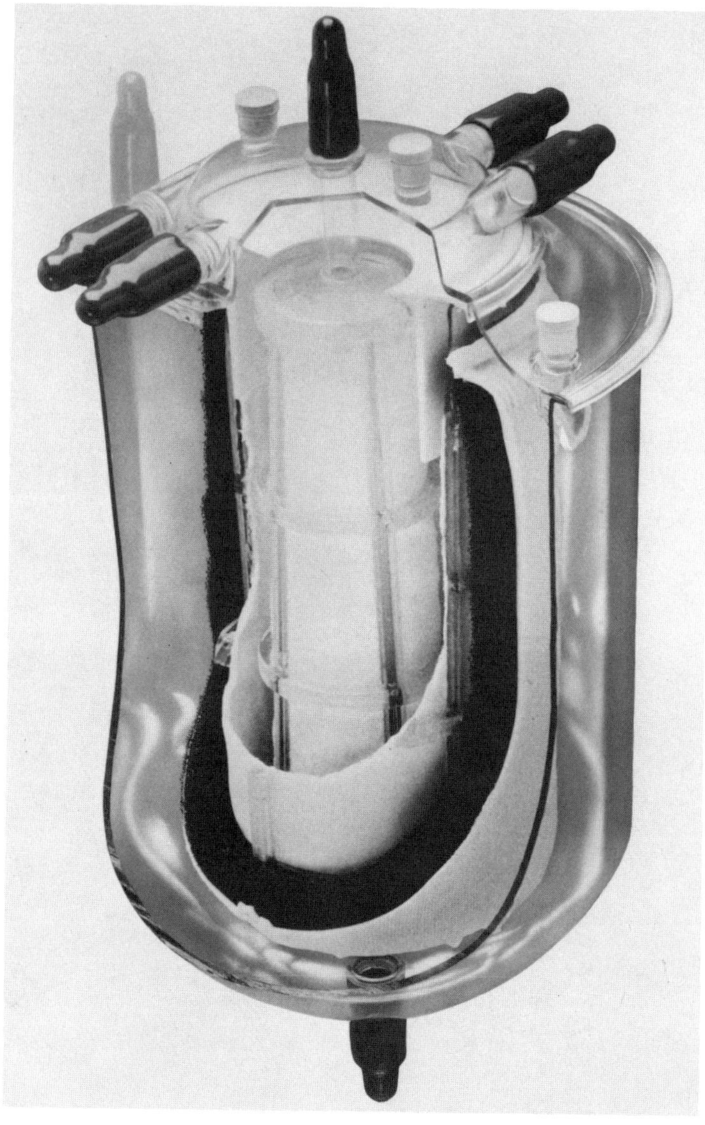

Figure 6.2 Most cardiotomy reservoirs contain both depth-type and screen-type filters. (Courtesy of Bard Cardiosurgery Division, Billerica, Massachusetts.)

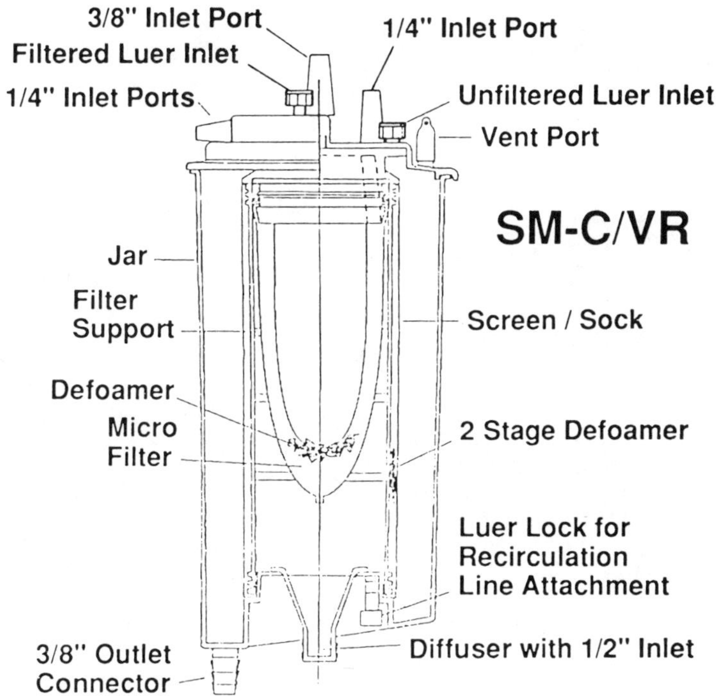

Figure 6.3 A hardshell venous reservoir with an integral cardiotomy reservoir to be used with a membrane oxygenator. Cross section. (Courtesy of SCIMED Life Systems, Inc., Minneapolis, Minnesota.)

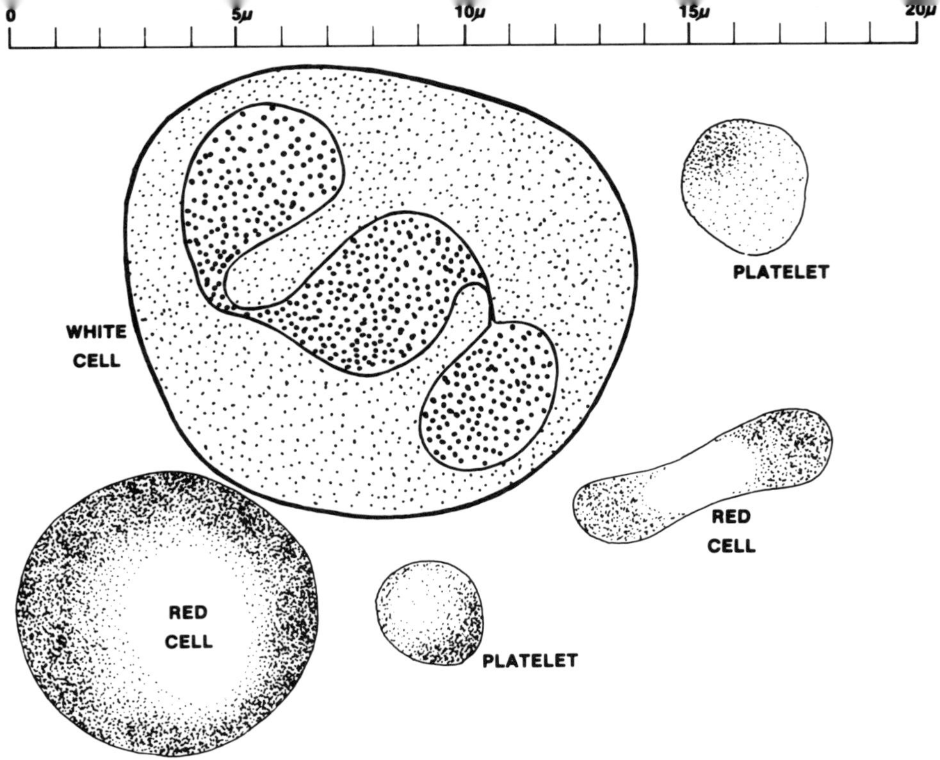

Figure 6.4 White cells, red cells, and platelets are shown in relative size on a micron scale.

the leukocytes who chemically detect the dead cell and treat it as if it were a foreign protein. In the extracorporeal circuit, however, the dead red cell membranes may clump together, at which time they must be removed by a filter. Platelets, although relatively small, also have a tendency to clump together in numbers that can produce a particle large enough to form a microembolus. This clumping, called "aggregation," must also be removed by the filtration system.

The ideal filter should have a negligible hydraulic resistance to blood flow and should cause a minimum amount of blood trauma. It should have a large enough surface area so that it can still filter effectively when it is partially plugged with filtered debris. However, the best size and type of extracorporeal bloodstream filter is still a matter of debate among the experts.

From early in the history of cardiopulmonary bypass, filters have been placed in a final position just prior to the return of oxygenated blood to the patient's body (Figure 6.5). These filters have ranged in filtering capacity from 20 to 125 microns. Most of the filters have been screen-types. Present day in-line filters are used not only to remove solid particles from the extracorporeal circuit, but also to remove gaseous micro-emboli produced by the circuit. Many perfusionists prefer to use the in-line arterial filter as a primary safety device to prevent gross air embolization (Figure 6.6). If the oxygenator is accidentally emptied of blood, air may be vented back to the oxygenator instead of being infused into the patient's arterial circulation.

Filters are also placed in the cardiotomy reservoir to filter out debris returned from the hand-held cardiotomy suction system. These filters are capable of removing lipid particles, fibrin, and platelet clumps.

Filters are also used in a recirculation line before bypass. Called "pre-bypass filters," they remove particulate matter (especially manufacturing residue) from the extracorporeal circuit (Figure 6.7).

Filters are also used to filter bacteria from the gas before it enters the oxygenator. This kind of filter must

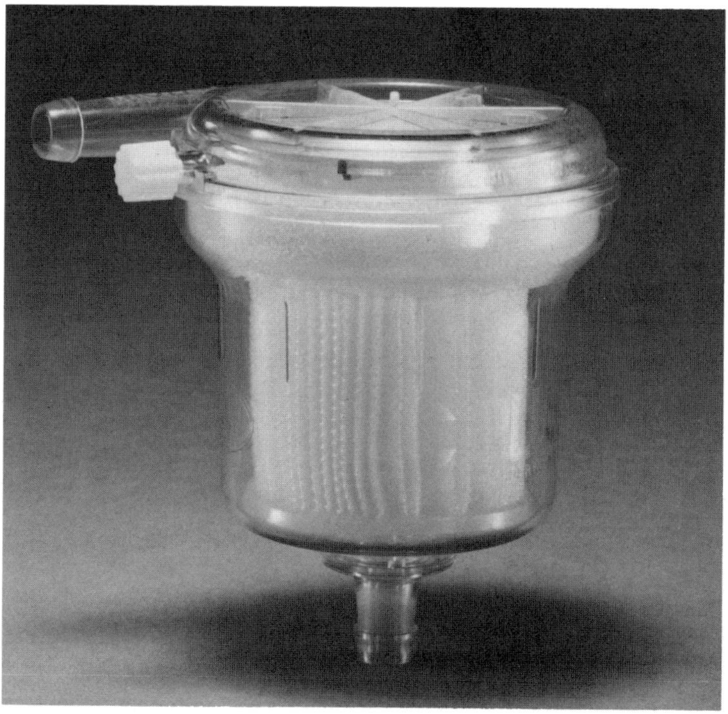

Figure 6.5 A modern, inline, arterial blood filter. (Courtesy of Pall Biomedical Products Corporation, Glen Cove, New York.)

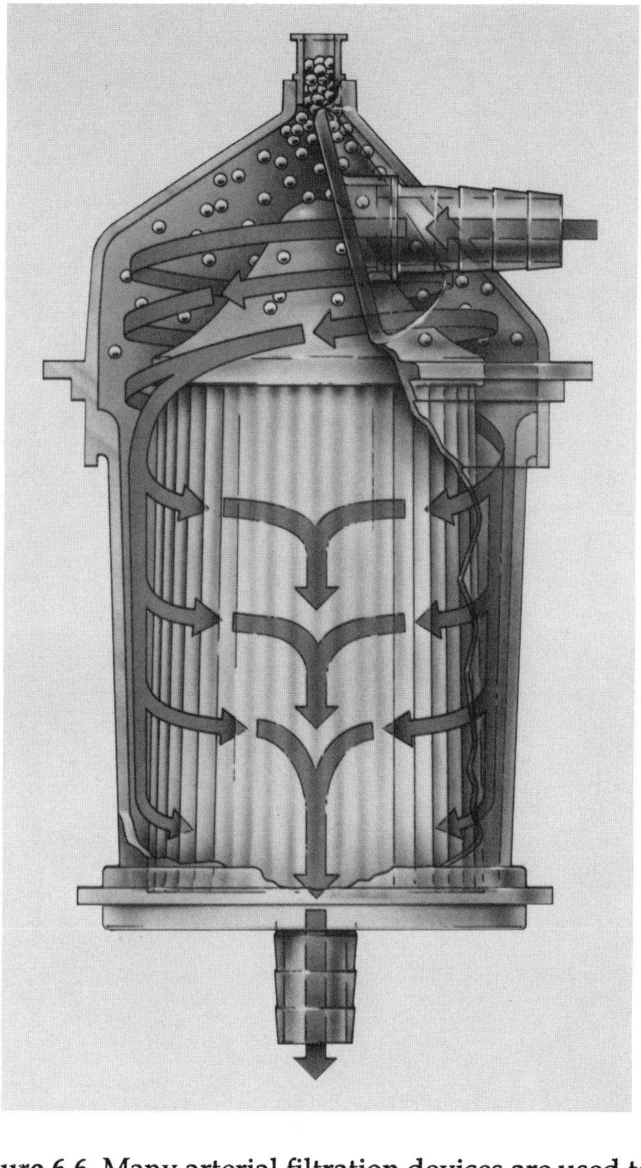

Figure 6.6 Many arterial filtration devices are used to prevent gross air embolization. (Courtesy of Bard Cardiosurgery Division, Billerica, Massachusetts.)

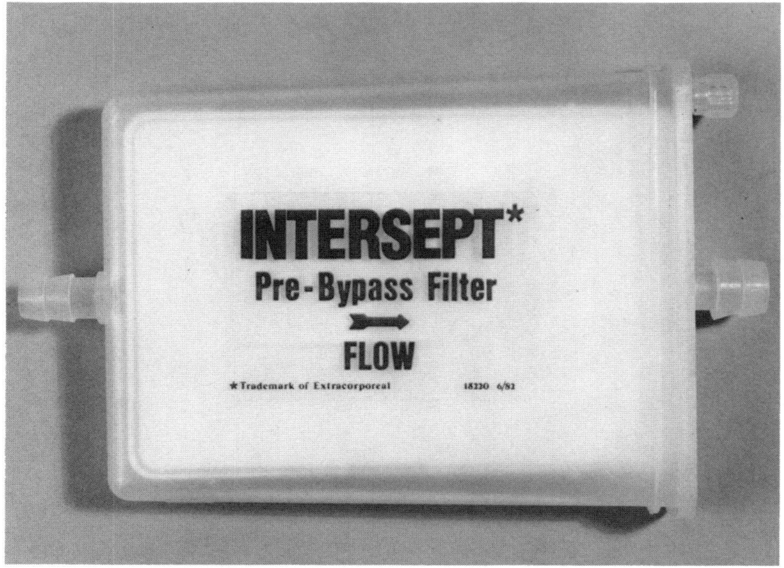

Figure 6.7 Filters are also used to remove solid debris from the circuit prior to bypass. (Courtesy of Johnson & Johnson Company, King-of-Prussia, Pennsylvania.)

remove microbes as small as .2 microns.

Heat Exchangers

Cells produce heat as a by-product of their metabolism. The heat produced by body cells is either eliminated to the external environment or is stored in body tissue. In "warm-blooded" (homothermous) animals, body temperature can be affected by external temperature extremes, physical exercise, or by some kinds of emotional stress and disease conditions. "Normal body temperature" is a measurement of body temperature in a healthy individual who is not exposed to any thermal stresses. Normal body temperature taken rectally is 37° Centigrade. Taken orally, it is 36.7° Centigrade. The human body employs an internal thermal regulatory system to conserve or to reduce body heat. This thermal regulation is accomplished by vasodilatation or vasoconstriction, which in turn, changes the blood flow patterns to the organ systems. Various organ systems, including the skin, exhibit temperature variations within the body.

Heat exchangers are used in extracorporeal blood circuits to maintain blood temperature at a desired level (Figure 6.8). The temperature of the perfused blood then maintains the body tissues at the predetermined level (Figure 6.9).

The position of the heat exchanger in the extracorporeal circuit has long been a concern of perfusion physiologists. It has been determined that the best place for the heat exchanger is on the venous side of the circuit. During the rewarming phase of hypothermic perfusion, bubbles can be liberated from the blood if rewarming occurs too rapidly. To prevent this problem, many perfusionists maintain the difference between blood temperature and the water temperature in the exchanger at a level not to exceed 10-12° C. It is also possible to overheat the blood by exposing it to too high a temperature. Blood flowing through a heat exchanger should not be exposed to temperatures higher than 45° Centigrade. Many perfusionists use 42° C as their maximum safe water temperature during rewarming. Stationary blood

BLOOD/WATER HEAT EXCHANGER

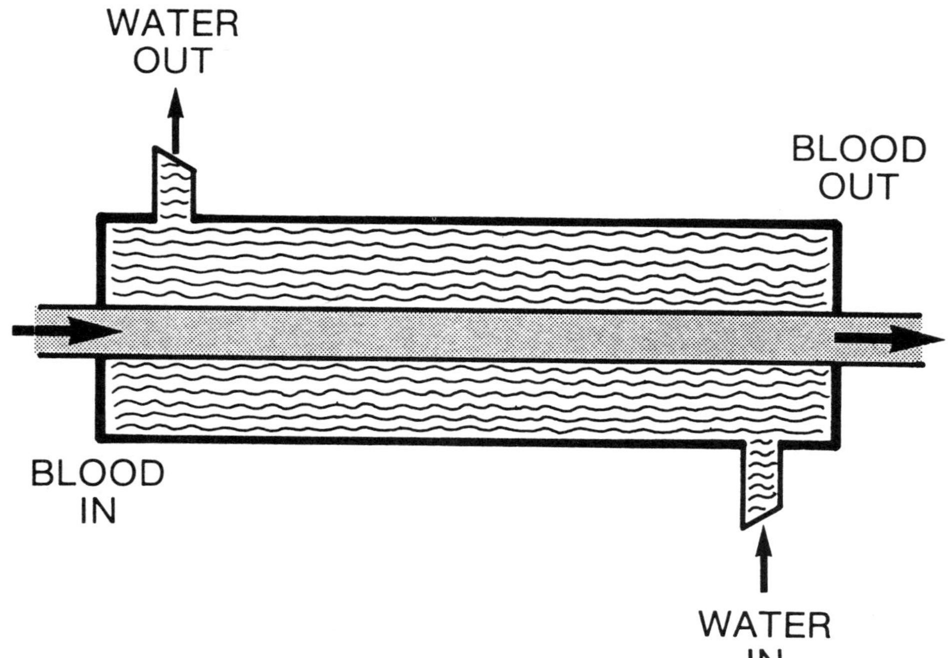

Figure 6.8 Heat exchangers are used to regulate the temperature of the blood. The temperature is controlled from the heart-lung machine's console by the perfusionist.

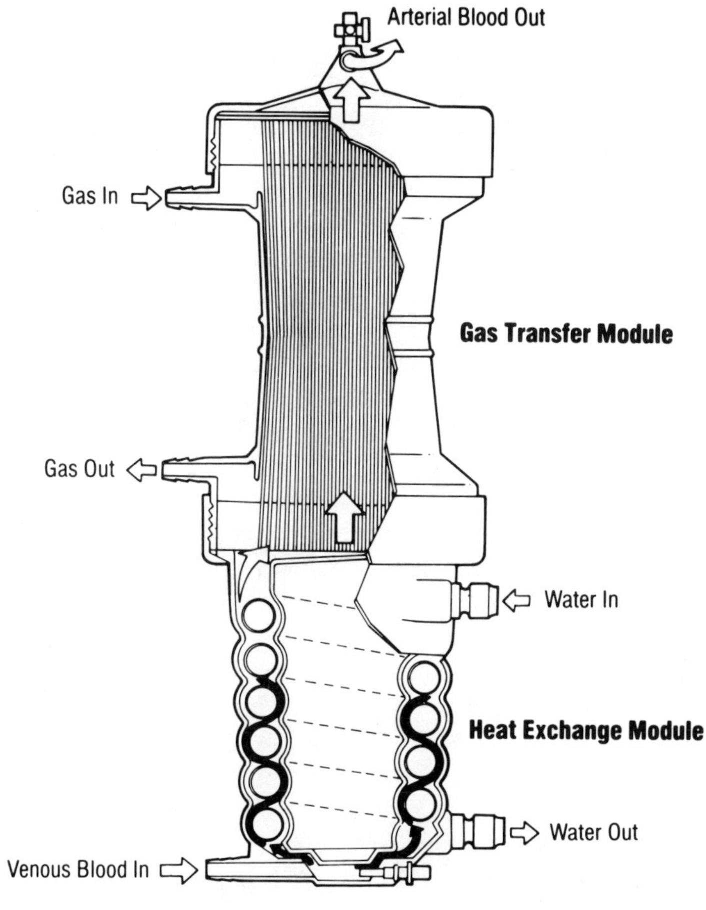

Figure 6.9 Most artificial lungs have internal heat exchangers. (Courtesy of Baxter Healthcare Corporation, Bentley Laboratories Division, Irvine, California.)

should not be exposed to temperatures much above normal body temperature—38-39° C. Blood damage, such as a lysis of the blood cells and protein denaturization, can occur at higher temperatures (Figure 6.10).

Cardiotomy Suction System

Even though a patient is on total cardiopulmonary bypass, some blood may return to the heart chambers. Blood returns to the right heart from the coronary arteries through the coronary sinus. Blood which returns to the left heart may be from the bronchial venous drainage into the left atrium. Although blood returning to the heart through a competent aortic valve should be minimal, blood will often leak in retrograde fashion through an aortic valve into the left ventricle because of aortic valvular insufficiency.

In order to clear the blood from the heart chambers, a system has been devised called the "cardiotomy suction system." Cardiotomy suctioning is used to return blood to the extracorporeal circuit through the cardiotomy (opening into the heart) (Figure 6.11). This system is also used during closed heart procedures, such as coronary artery grafting, to prevent the ventricular chambers from overdistending. An over-distended heart chamber can cause irreversible stretching damage to the heart muscle.

Blood is returned from the surgical field either by a hand-held cardiotomy suction tip or by a catheter placed into one of the heart cavities. Usually, a catheter is placed in the left ventricular heart cavity by inserting the catheter through the superior pulmonary vein and on through the mitral valve. Alternately, a catheter can also be inserted directly into the left ventricle through a stab wound made in the apex of the heart.

At times, there may be massive amounts of surgical bleeding, so the cardiotomy suction system must be capable of carrying a large blood flow (Figures 6.12 and 6.13). Primary requirements for a cardiotomy suction system are that (1) the system should handle blood gently, and (2) that it be capable of removing air from the blood that may enter

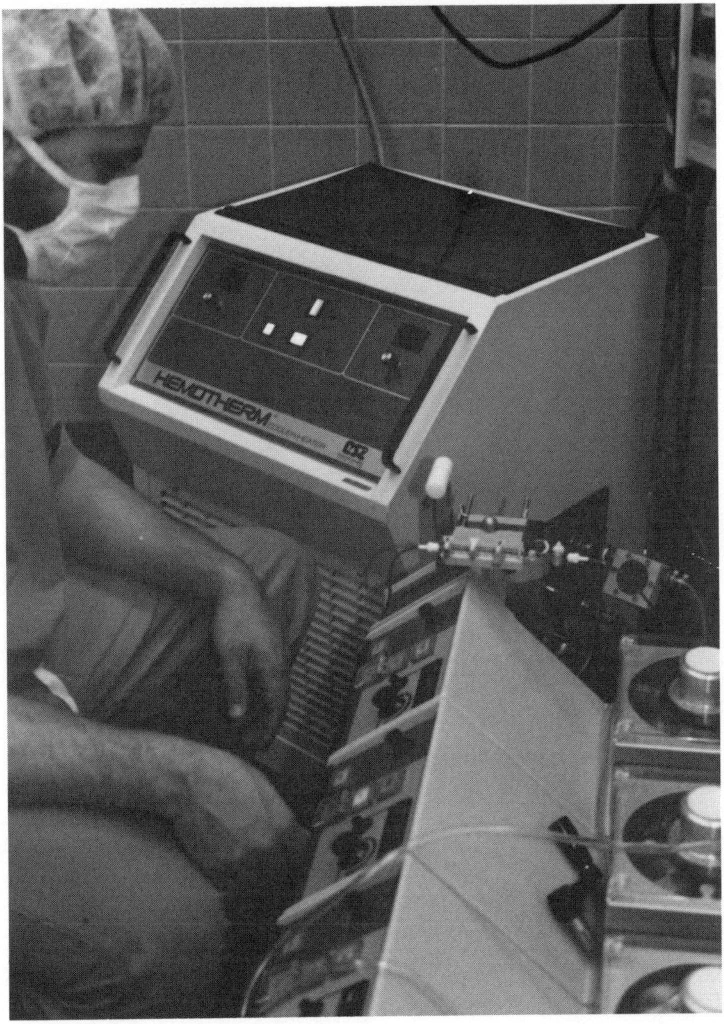

Figure 6.10 The temperature control systemat the perfusionist's left controls the temperature of the water, which, in turn, controls the temperature of the patient's blood. (Courtesy of Cincinnati Sub-Zero Products, Inc., Cincinnati, Ohio.)

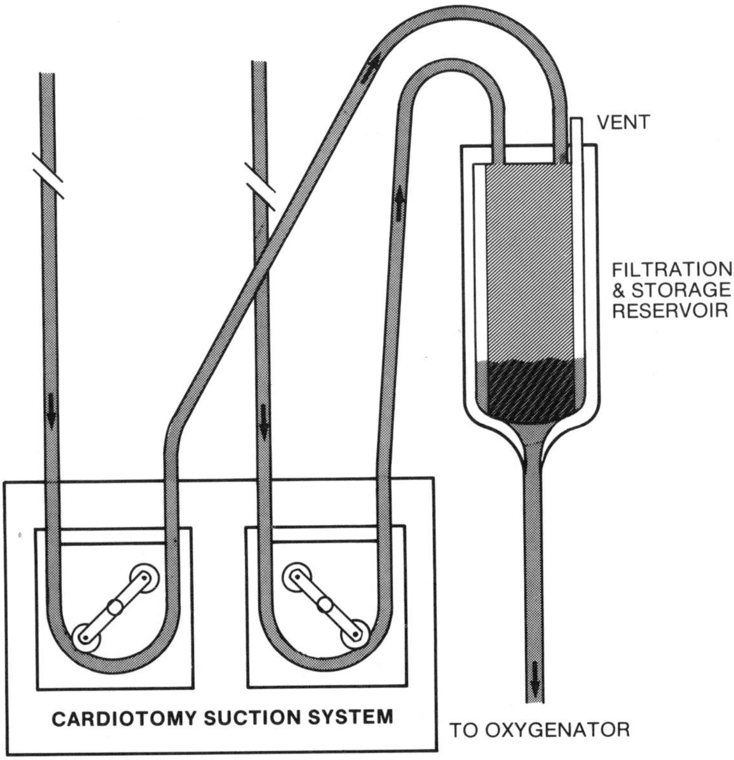

Figure 6.11 A cardiotomy suction system returns blood which might otherwise be lost or discarded to the heart-lung machine .

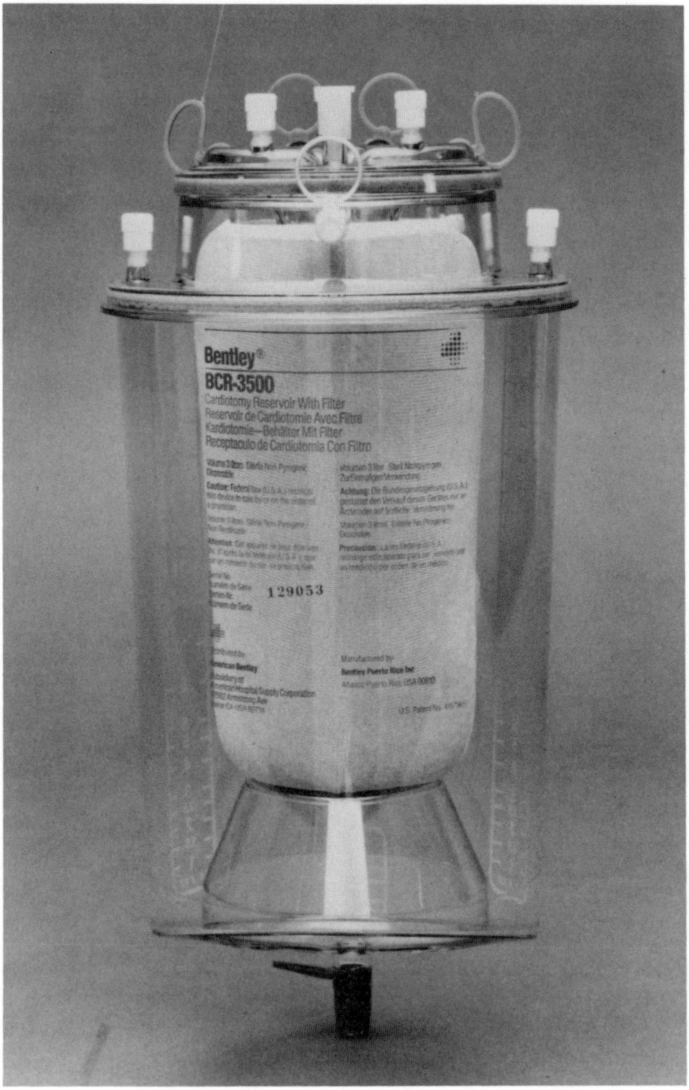

Figure 6.12 Some cardiotomy reservoirs have large volume capacity. This reservoir is designed to hold 3,500 cc. (Courtesy of Baxter Healthcare Corporation, Bentley Laboratories Division, Irvine, California.)

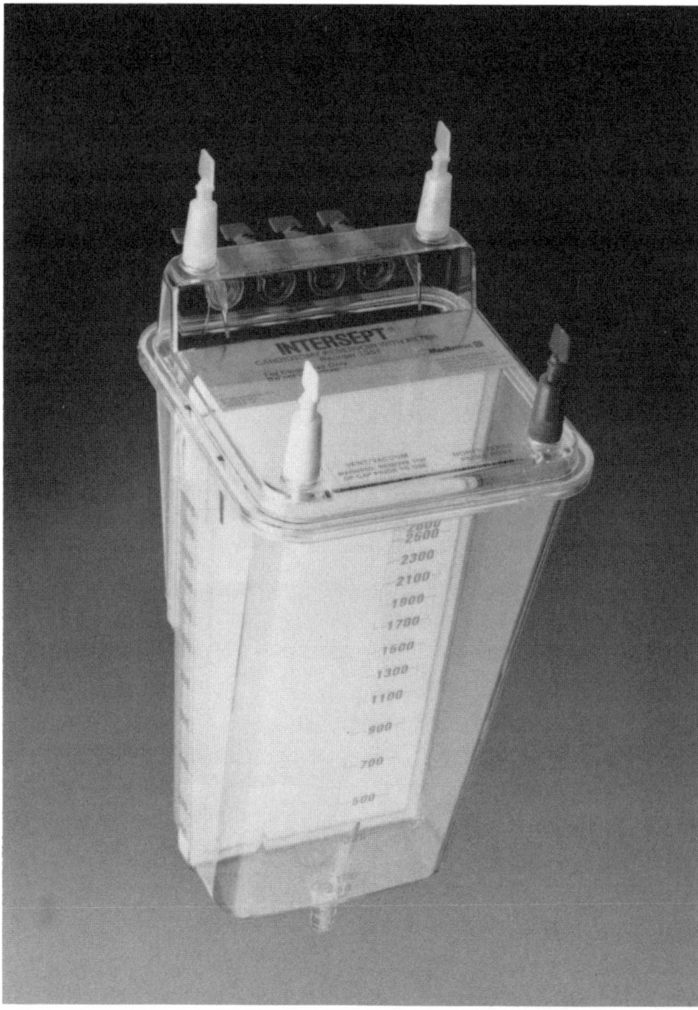

Figure 6.13 The cardiotomy suction system must be able to handle large blood flows in situations when blood floods the surgical field. (Courtesy of Medtronic Blood Systems, Inc., Anaheim, California.)

at the surgical site. Most cardiotomy suction system reservoirs have a defoaming chamber similar to the ones used in bubble oxygenation systems. Many state-of-the-art cardiotomy reservoirs also filter blood—down to the 20 micron range.

Some oxygenation systems have been manufactured that have built-in cardiotomy reservoirs. Proponents of these systems claim that there is less blood trapped ("held-up") in the cardiotomy reservoir and that this kind of system is less expensive. Perhaps one disadvantage of this kind of system is that if the cardiotomy reservoir becomes plugged, it cannot be changed. Too, one cannot electively store blood in the reservoir. However, many open-heart teams successfully use oxygenation systems with integral cardiotomy reservoirs.

It has been found that cardiotomy suction systems cause increased blood trauma during cardiopulmonary bypass. By reducing the amount of blood returned to a cardiotomy suction system and by reducing the speed at which blood is returned, excessive blood trauma can be kept to a minimum. However, there have been some studies which indicate that blood spilled from the cardiotomy into the pericardial sac is very rapidly hemolyzed. This hemolytic activity seems to be chemical rather than mechanical in nature. It has also been noted that the blood can withstand increased amounts of positive pressure, but that it is very susceptible to damage under very slight negative pressures.

SECTION III
TECHNIQUES & PROBLEMS

PATHOPHYSIOLOGY OF CARDIOPULMONARY BYPASS

Chapter Seven

Blood Trauma

Extracorporeal circulation produces many deviations from normal body physiology. For example, all extracorporeal circuits traumatize the blood to some extent. When blood plasma is exposed to foreign surface areas, denaturization of plasma proteins takes place. That is to say, plasma proteins, which occur in long chains of rather large molecules, physically change their geometric structure. It is also known that some surfaces absorb protein molecules while other surfaces do not. In any case, however, all surfaces to which blood is exposed should be highly polished to prevent as much absorption and turbulence as possible (Figures 7.1 and 7.2). Denaturization of plasma proteins also takes place during blood-gas interface, such as the blood-gas interface used in bubble oxygenation (Figure 7.3). This denaturization of plasma proteins is important because the factors responsible for the blood clotting mechanism are found in the plasma. Abnormal blood clotting can occur if the clotting factors are eliminated or if excessive hemodilution occurs, such as excessive hemodilution of the plasma by a crystalloid prime.

Measurement of free hemoglobin in the plasma is commonly used as an indication of the amount of blood trauma in an extracorporeal circuit. As we mentioned before, red cells are biconcave discs which are carried in the liquid plasma suspension. The red cells' membranes are very thin and therefore are susceptible to rupture by mechanical means, by excessive osmotic pressure, or by lysis

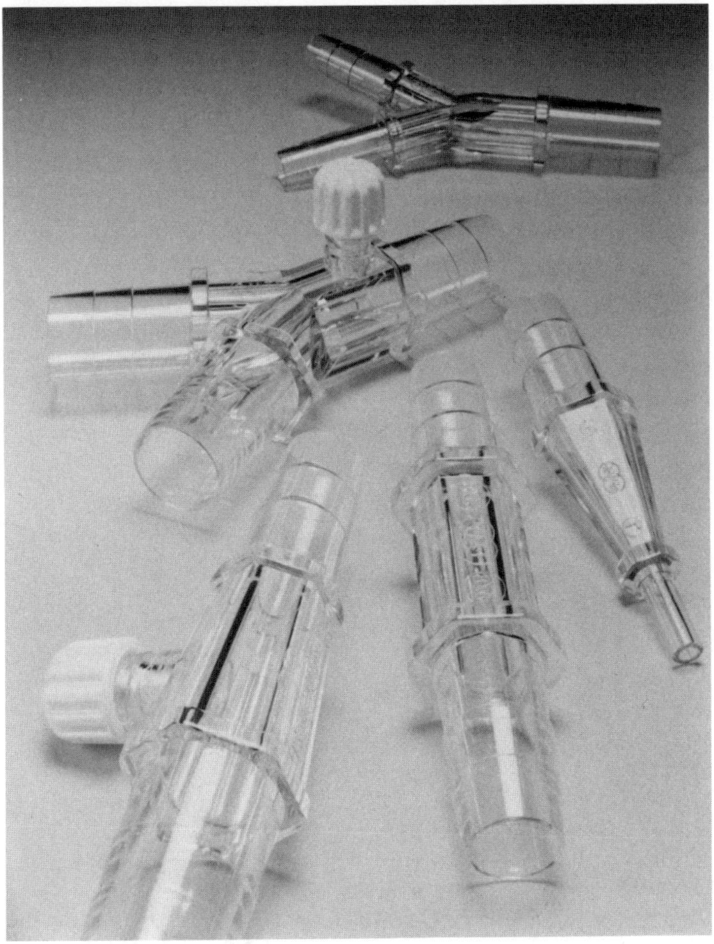

Figure 7.1 Extracorporeal blood connectors must have highly polished surfaces to avoid excessive blood damage. (Courtesy of Norton-Texas Medical Products, Houston, Texas.)

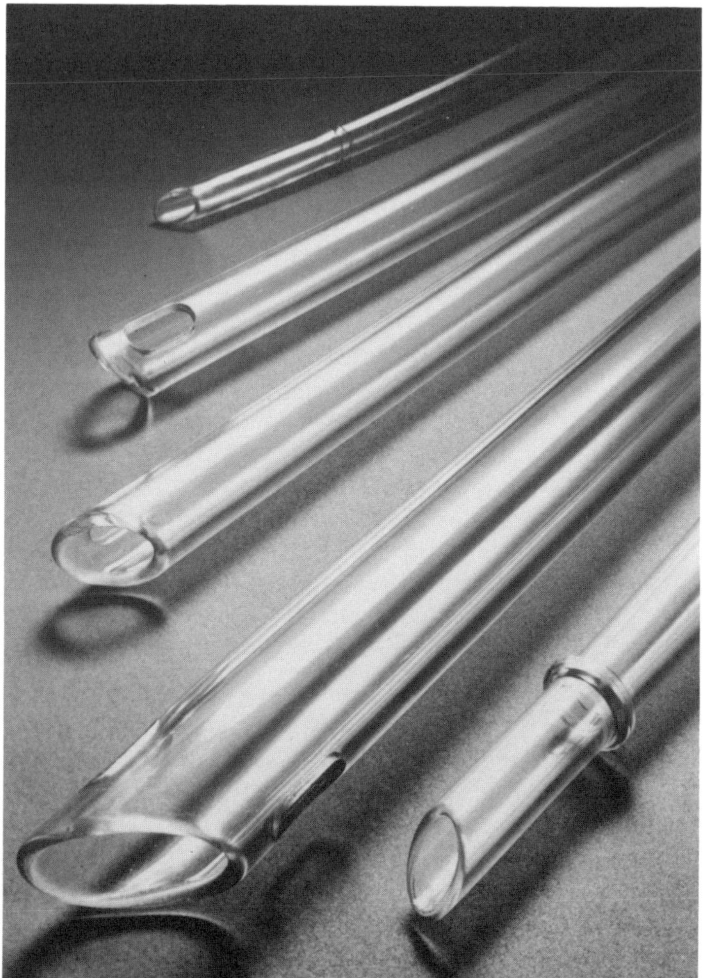

Figure 7.2 Cannulas are the most restrictive points in an extracorporeal circuit. (Courtesy of Norton-Texas Medical Products, Houston, Texas.)

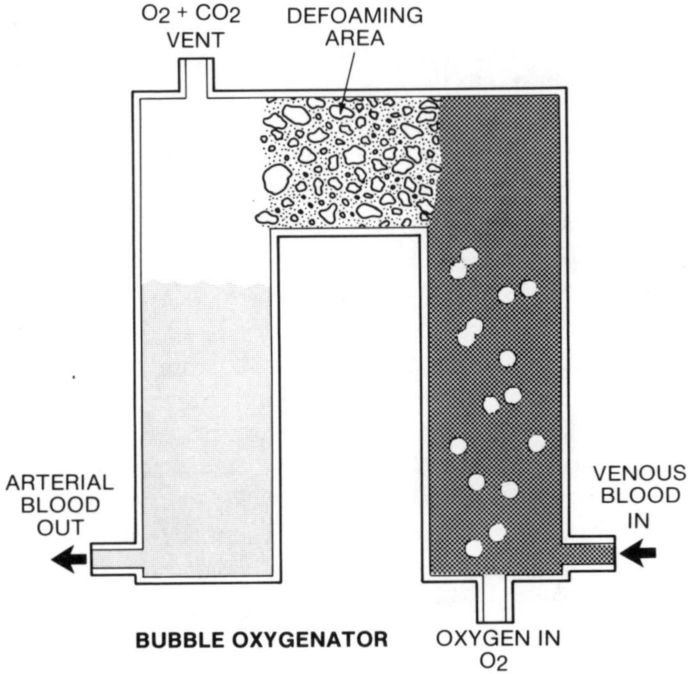

Figure 7.3 Direct blood gas interface is responsible for plasma protein denaturization when a bubble-type oxygenator is used.

resulting from age (red cells have an approximate 120 day life cycle). In the laboratory, the amount of free hemoglobin remaining in the plasma after ruptured red cells have been centrifuged from a blood sample gives an indication of the amount of hemolysis caused by blood trauma. Too, levels of free hemoglobin in the plasma are generally elevated in a time-related phenomenon. The longer the period of extracorporeal perfusion, the more hemolysis occurs. In an active, living organism, however, damaged free hemoglobin in the plasma is eliminated by the kidneys and by the reticular endothelial system. Therefore, if one wished to investigate the exact amount of blood trauma caused by a particular extracorporeal circuit, one would have to look at the circuit in question by means of an *in vitro* or "bench test" method. In other words, some kind of "body" would have to be constructed in which the circulation bypassed the kidneys and reticuloendothelial system. Normal values for plasma-free hemoglobin are from 0-5 mg per 100 milliliters of blood.

Let's examine blood trauma in more detail. Blood normally flows through tubes (blood vessels) in a streamlined fashion. The blood flow's greatest velocity takes place in the center of the vessel. Slower velocities occur near or against the inside walls of the vessel because of the frictional resistance to blood flow. This flow, consisting of layers of blood with varying velocities ranging from the center to the sides of the vessel, is called "laminar flow." "Turbulent" or "non-streamlined" blood flow occurs when the walls of a blood vessel are narrowed or obstructed. Turbulent blood flow is associated with blood trauma (Figure 7.4).

Another mechanical cause of blood trauma can be the "jetting" effect of oxygen into the blood, mentioned earlier. "Jetting" is caused, you may remember, by excessive gas flows in a bubble oxygenator. Excessive heating of the blood in a heat exchanger can also cause damage to the red cells.

Extremely high osmotic pressure can cause massive hemolysis. Such a problem can occur when water, in the form of priming and other solutions, is added to the extra-

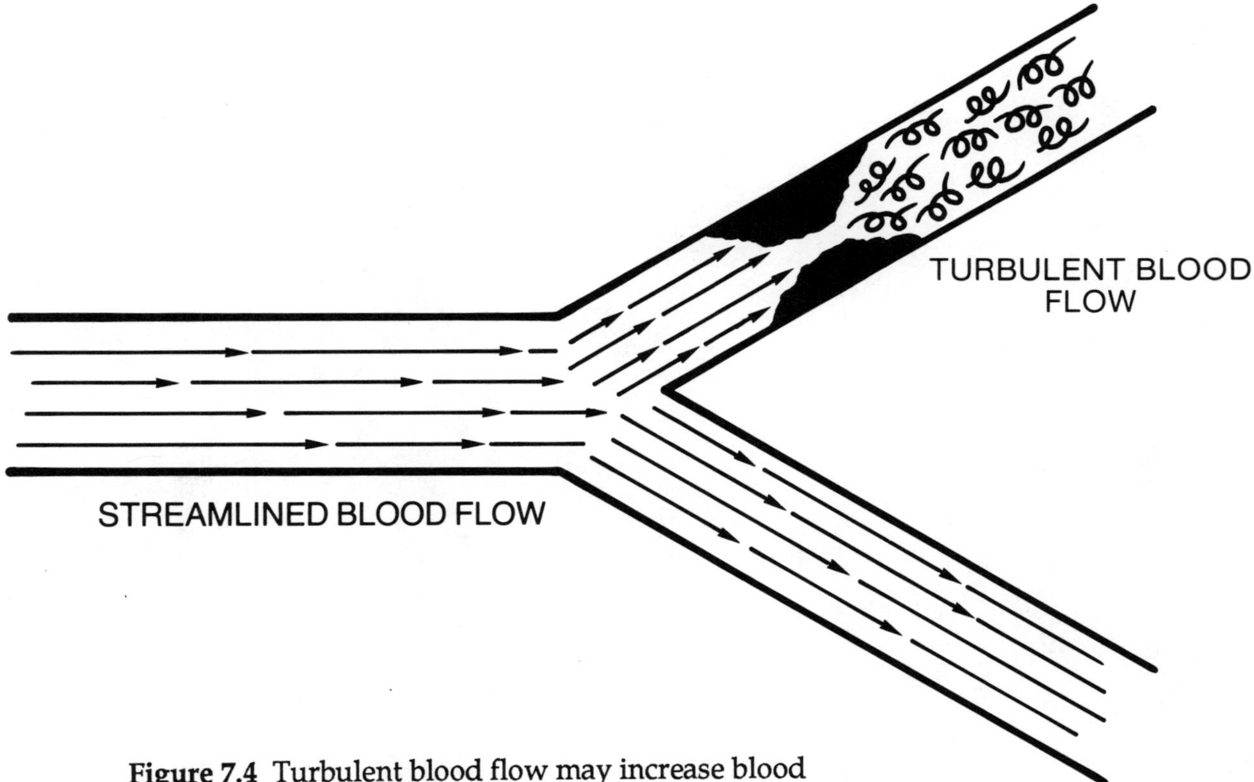

Figure 7.4 Turbulent blood flow may increase blood trauma.

corporeal circuit. The isotonicity of such solutions must be closely controlled (from 290-310 milliosmols) to prevent osmotic trauma. Accidental rupture of a heat exchanger with a resulting water leak into the blood can also cause massive hemolysis.

We have mentioned blood trauma in association with damage to the erythrocytes. Trauma can also occur to the plate-shaped thrombocytes (platelets), which are also in the plasma suspension. Thrombocytes react to foreign surface areas by adhering to those surfaces. As more and more thrombocytes adhere to a surface, they can aggregate, forming a potential embolus. As they clump together, they may also be removed from the circulating blood by the filtration system of the extracorporeal circuit. Without an adequate number of platelets in the blood, coagulation cannot be restored at the conclusion of perfusion. It is extremely important, then, to monitor heparin levels carefully during extracorporeal circulation in order not to activate the clotting mechanism (Figure 7.5). The clotting process has been described as a series of "cascading" events, each of which uses up chemicals necessary for clotting to occur. Once these chemicals are used up, there are no more immediately available. It may be important to note here that the thrombocyte count decreases at the start of bypass and then gradually returns to normal levels in the post-operative period—mostly due to hemodilution of the blood.

The effects of extracorporeal blood trauma on white blood cells is not as well documented as those with erythrocytes and thrombocytes. Damage to the white blood cells decreases their ability to fight disease.

Our immune system, the mechanism that fights off and protects our bodies from infection, is made up of leukocytes in combination with a series of complex proteins in the blood plasma that are called "complement." Normally, the complement is inactive until the body is invaded by disease organisms or suffers trauma. When these exposures occur, the complement is activated, causing an interaction with normal blood cells which may alter their normal

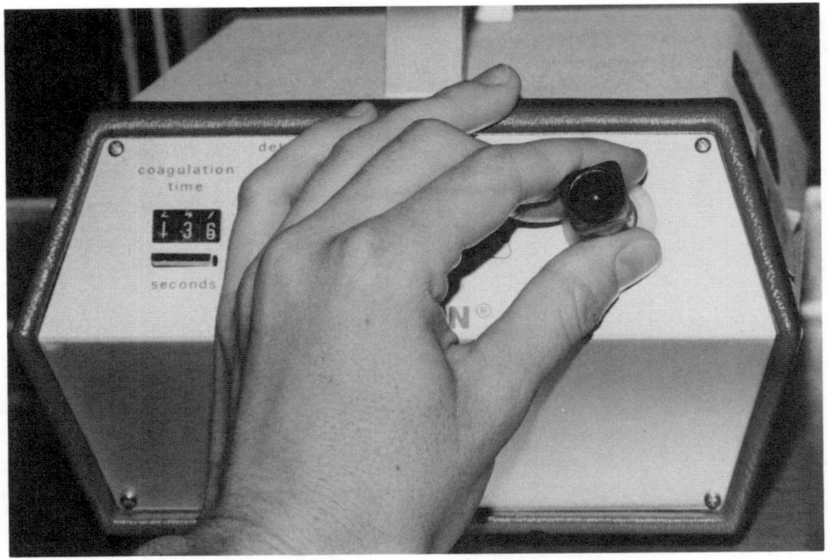

Figure 7.5 Taken during cardiopulmonary bypass, activated clotting time (ACT) is a measure of activated blood coagulation time expressed in seconds.

function. When this cascading kind of interaction occurs, the process is called "complement activation," and the process works to the body's advantage.

However, in some instances, when blood is exposed to some foreign surface areas, such as occurs in extracorporeal circulation, complement activation may be triggered prematurely, causing detrimental effects to the body. Premature complement activation can alter the immune system's ability to ward off disease. Many factors have been identified that activate the complement system. For example, direct blood-to-gas interface, such as occurs within bubble-type oxygenators, may trigger complement activation. Certain drugs which are recognized as foreign proteins by the immune system may trigger complement activation. For example, protamine sulphate, which is normally administered at the conclusion of cardiopulmonary bypass to reverse the action of heparin, an anticoagulant, has been identified as an activator. Certain synthetic materials, mainly nylon and cellophane, can activate the system when the complement comes in contact with these substances on the surfaces of the extracorporeal circuit. Again, the immune system recognizes these surfaces as foreign materials, thereby triggering the activation system.

One consequence of premature complement activation may be a condition called "post-perfusion syndrome" or "post-pump lung." This condition alters the pulmonary circulation and may result in pulmonary hemorrhage, and ultimately to pulmonary edema. Another consequence of premature activation may be a migration of leukocytes to the pulmonary capillaries, impairing pulmonary function. Other organ dysfunctions may occur, such as impaired cardiac and renal function.

One other very important result of premature complement activation is that the chemicals involved in complement activation are depleted, impairing the body's capability to fight disease on an on-going basis.

All extracorporeal circuits cause some blood trauma. Typically, the extent of blood damage is usually an acceptable amount for the few hours that it takes to accomplish the surgical repair. However, if excessive blood trauma does take place, some possible clinical symptoms are: blind spots on the retina, impairment of the clotting mechanism, impairment of the complement activation system, and other clinical evidence of microembolization.

Trauma to the blood during cardiopulmonary bypass can be minimized by limiting the time that the patient is on bypass, by paying meticulous attention to the amount of cardiotomy suction used during the surgical procedure, and by ensuring that the extracorporeal circuit is composed entirely of biocompatible materials.

Improper Venous Return

Approximately 80% of the total blood volume of an adult is contained in the venous and capillary networks. It is not surprising, then, that small changes in venous pressure can be reflected by large changes in blood volume. During cardiopulmonary bypass, venous cannulation can introduce a significant alteration in blood flow, which, in turn, results in altered venous pressure (Figure 7.6). Small changes in blood volume can dramatically affect the flow of blood returned to the oxygenator. To reduce these changes in pressure and volume as much as possible, the selection of catheter size and the positioning of the catheter(s) within the low pressure venous system must be considered with care (Figure 7.7). The catheter(s) must be large enough to drain the central veins adequately, yet be small enough to avoid interference with right atrial filling during partial bypass. Venous drainage should not be mechanically obstructed by manipulation of the heart for long periods of time, and the venous blood flow should be totally diverted to the heart-lung machine. Ideally, venous blood should not pool in the heart and lungs, thus flooding the surgical field and obstructing the surgeon's view. Since return to the right atrium is by way of two separate return conduits, the superior and inferior vena cavae, it is possible to obstruct one venous vascular bed and not the other.

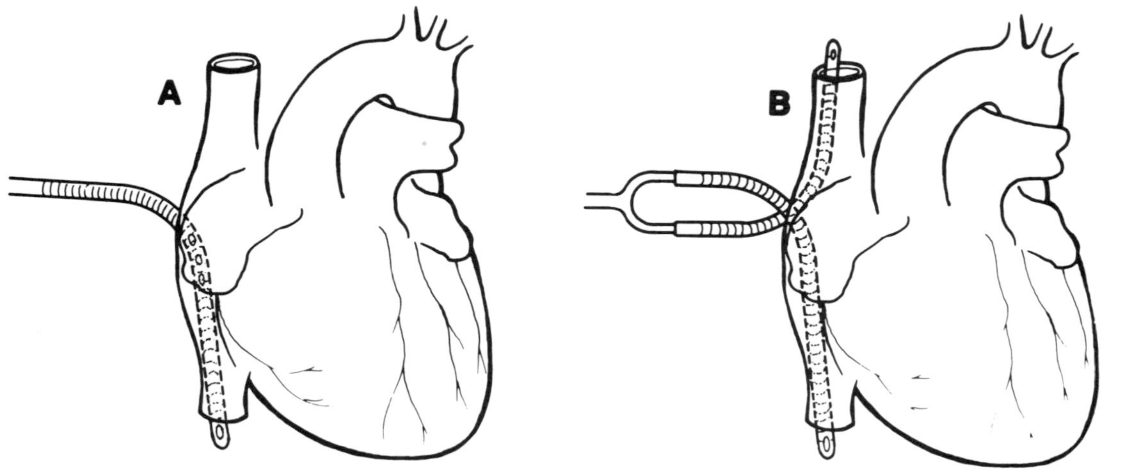

Figure 7.6 (A) Dual stage cannula. (B) Individual cannulation of the inferior and superior vena cavae.

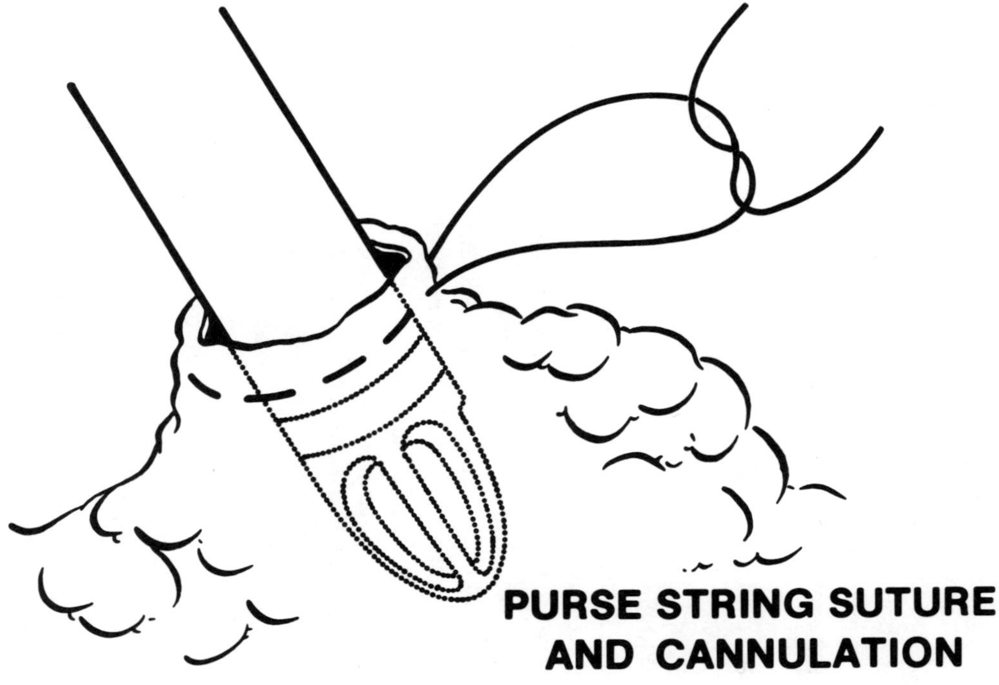

Figure 7.7 Venous cannulas are inserted into heart cavities through incisions (atriotomies) controlled by purse string sutures.

Improper venous return can lead to a number of problems. First, obstructed venous return will reduce the total blood flow, and metabolic acidosis will result because of the deficit. Second, a rapid decrease in venous return to an oxygenator without a corresponding decrease in output can accidentally empty the oxygenator (Figure 7.8). This will result in an infusion of gas emboli into the arterial circulation.

A third problem involving improper venous return is more complex—excessive hemodilution. If the venous catheter(s) is partially obstructed, such as occurs when the surgeon must lift and manipulate the heart, the effects of the obstruction can sometimes be compensated by the addition of fluids to the circuit. However, this attempt to solve one problem may result in the creation of other problems. Fluid overload during cardiopulmonary bypass may be defined as the transfusion of fluids in excess of the volume needed to maintain a safe operating level in the extracorporeal circuit. Fluid overload by using crystalloidal solutions (such as lactated Ringer's and 5% dextrose in H_2O) can increase tissue edema as fluid accumulates in the cellular interstitial spaces. Fluid overload or hemodilution can also increase diuresis, thus increasing the possibility of hypokalemia (abnormally low serum potassium). Hypokalemia can trigger cardiac arrhythmias. Drugs may be lost through excessive diuresis. Hemodilution also reduces the oxygen-carrying capacity. Reduced oxygen-carrying capacity of the blood in conjunction with reduced perfusion flow is a double insult to cellular metabolism. Hemodilution can also reduce the clotting factors in the blood in an amount that is directly proportional to the amount of hemodilution.

A fourth problem caused by obstructed venous return is a corresponding high venous pressure, which, in turn, exerts an excessively high capillary pressure. Excessively high capillary pressure results in a shift of fluid into the cellular interstitial spaces. If this fluid shift is allowed to continue, the resultant profound tissue edema can cause severe organ dysfunction.

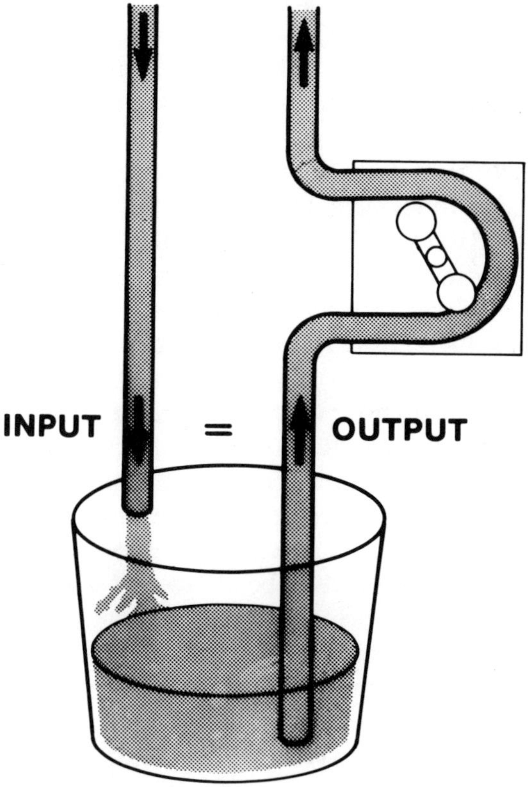

Figure 7.8 If input does not equal output in a vented artificial lung, an arterial infusion of gas emboli may take place.

Sporadic changes in venous return to the heart-lung machine can cause a fifth problem—hemodynamic instability of the perfusion (Figure 7.9). During perfusion, peripheral vascular resistance increases with increased venous pressure. If the position of the venous catheter(s) is changed as a result of manipulation of the heart during the surgical procedure, venous return to the heart-lung machine can be changed rapidly. If tourniquets are not placed around the vena cavae, these changes become even more evident. Even more hemodynamic instability may result from manipulation of the heart if single right atrial cannulation is employed. Repeated shifts in blood volume between the patient and the heart-lung machine may lead to an unstable patient, and frequently to one who is pharmacologically over-treated as well.

A sixth problem involving impaired venous return concerns heat exchange. Reduced blood flow reduces the amount of heat transfer that takes place during extracorporeal heat exchange. As a result, both the rewarming and the cooling processes are slowed. Distribution of blood flow to various vascular beds may be altered by obstruction in venous return. Thus, various organs may not benefit from hypothermia during rapid bloodstream cooling and may not be effectively rewarmed during the rewarming phase of perfusion.

The last problem we will discuss concerning improper venous return involves a compromise of myocardial protection during heart surgery in which hypothermic cardioplegia is employed. A variety of methods are used during hypothermic cardioplegia to administer the cardioplegic solutions, to vent the heart, and to cannulate for venous return. A single right arterial cannula has become widely used for coronary artery surgery. The so-called "dual stage" venous catheter is also employed during aorto-coronary bypass grafting. Following cannulation, cardiopulmonary bypass is initiated, and the patient is usually cooled systemically. When the patient's temperature reaches a desired level, the aorta is cross-clamped, and cardioplegic

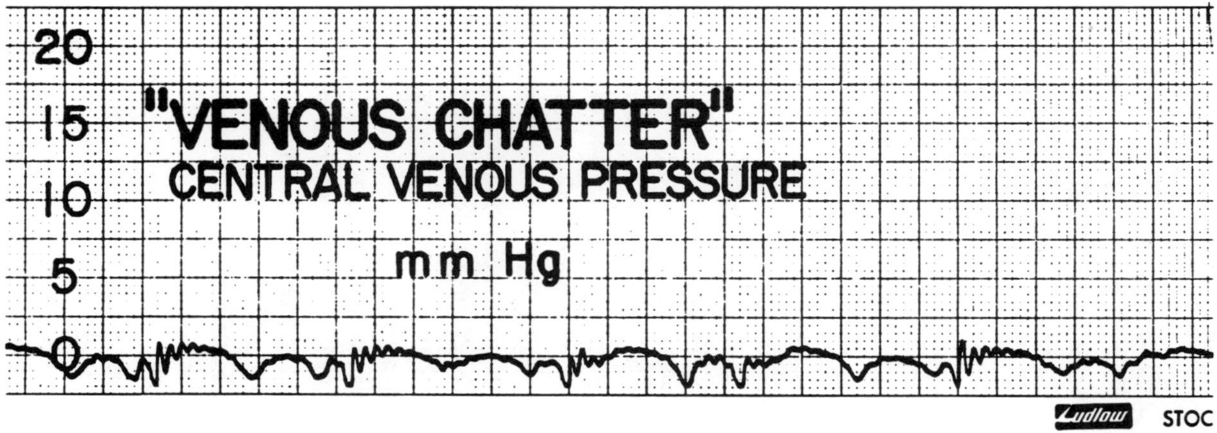

Figure 7.9 Venous pressure during heart-lung bypass may be below atmospheric pressure (zero on the vertical scale).

solution is infused into the aorta. The effectiveness of cardioplegia is judged by observing the cessation of electromechanical heart activity and by monitoring myocardial temperature, which should decrease. Elevated right atrial pressure (as can occur with obstructed venous return) can cause retrograde perfusion of the coronary sinus, resulting in myocardial rewarming and inadequate myocardial protection.

Arterial Infusion

The greatest pressures encountered in the human circulatory system are those generated in the left ventricle. With each ventricular contraction, the heart ejects blood into the arterial system with a force sufficient to maintain a mean arterial blood pressure in the range of 90 to 100 millimeters of mercury (90-100 mmHg). It is in this contractile phase, systole, that arterial pressure reaches its highest level. During the relaxation phase, diastole, blood pressure drops off to its lowest level. It is during diastole that the ventricle fills with blood to make ready for the next contraction. It is this pressure differential across the circulatory system from the aorta to the vena cava that is responsible for the driving force that moves blood. Many of the physical laws governing fluid motion can be applied to the hemodynamics of the cardiovascular system. However, as we mentioned before, blood is not a pure fluid, but rather is a complex, heterogeneous fluid of varying viscosity. Too, the tubes or vessels into which the heart ejects blood are not solid, nondistensible tubes but rather are soft and pliable. The cross sectional area of the arteries can also be changed by selective arterial constriction or dilation.

Blood is usually returned from the heart-lung machine to the patient in one of two sites (Figure 7.10). One site is the aortic arch, which is widely-used for open heart surgery. In this procedure, a purse-string suture is placed in the aorta, and an aortotomy is made. The arterial catheter (Figure 7.11) is placed through the purse-string suture and affixed to the suture. The other site for arterial infusion is

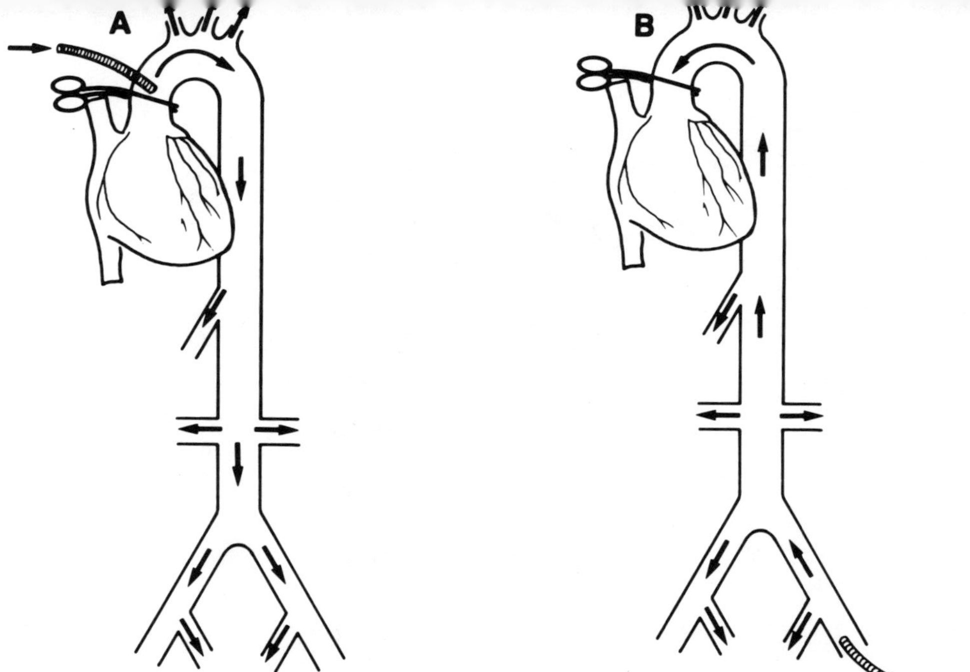

Figure 7.10 Cannulation sites for reinfusion of arterial blood: (A) Blood is returned into the arch of the aorta. (B) Blood is returned into the femoral artery.

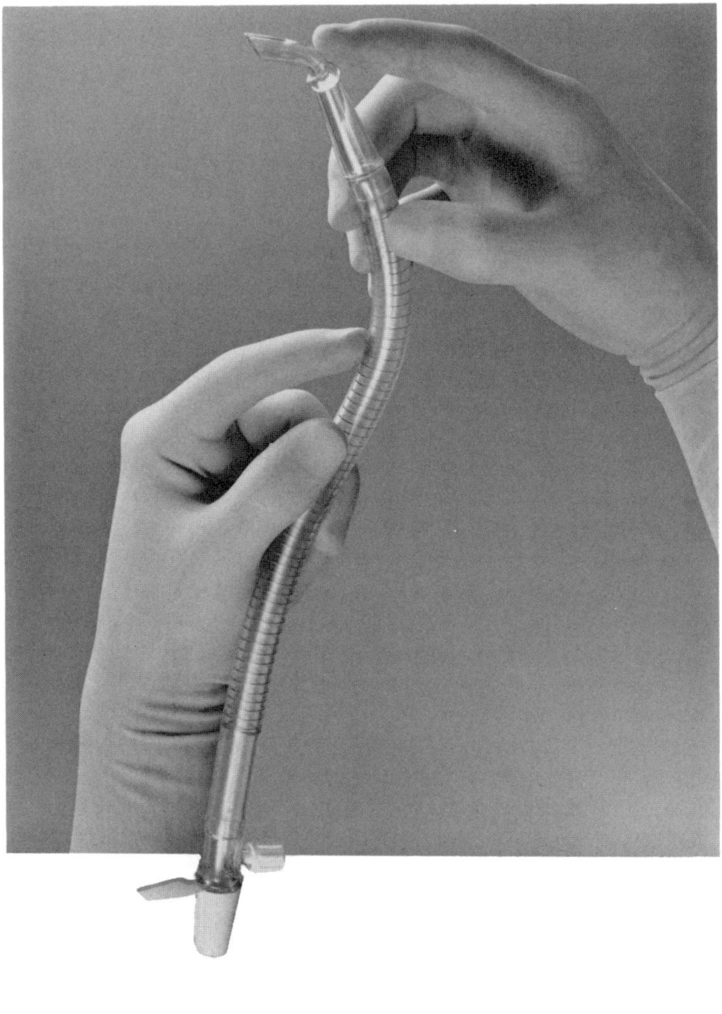

Figure 7.11 Aortic arch cannula. (Courtesy of Sarns, 3M Healthcare, Ann Arbor, Michigan.)

through the femoral arteries. In this case, blood which flows into the aorta occurs mostly in a retrograde fashion; whereas most blood flow, when aortic cannulation is used, occurs in a normal flow path.

The highest pressures encountered in a heart-lung machine are near the outlet of the arterial pump. Arterial blood re-enters the circulatory system through a catheter that has a smaller cross-sectional area than the blood vessel into which the catheter is placed. It is important that the surgeon choose a catheter that is as large as is practical to insert into the arteriotomy in order to avoid high pressure gradients. High pressure gradients between the catheter and the receiving blood vessel are undesirable. For example, a high pressure gradient can create a slight back pressure behind the site of the catheter, causing cavitation. Cavitation, which is a partial vacuum created in a liquid, can liberate bubbles which, in turn, become potential emboli.

There are other problems caused by the smaller diameter of the arterial reentry catheter. To explain them, we must briefly review the anatomy of an artery. As you may remember, arteries are composed of three distinct tissue layers: the outer layer, or adventitia; the middle muscular layer, the media; and the endothelialized, innermost layer, the intima (Figure 7.12). During the insertion of the arterial cannula, it is possible for the surgeon to erroneously insert the catheter tip between the intima and the media instead of into the lumen of the artery. In this case, when arterial infusion is begun, an arterial dissection can occur—stripping away the intima, collapsing the lumen, and obstructing the blood flow. The perfusionist can usually diagnose the problem early in the perfusion by observing the pressure in the arterial line that runs from the outlet of the pump to the arterial cannulation site. In may be important to note here that arterial dissection can also occur as the result of arteriosclerotic disease and Marfan's syndrome.

Sometimes, a jetting effect occurs at the site of arterial reentry when using a small arterial cannula because this site becomes the most restrictive point in the extracorporeal

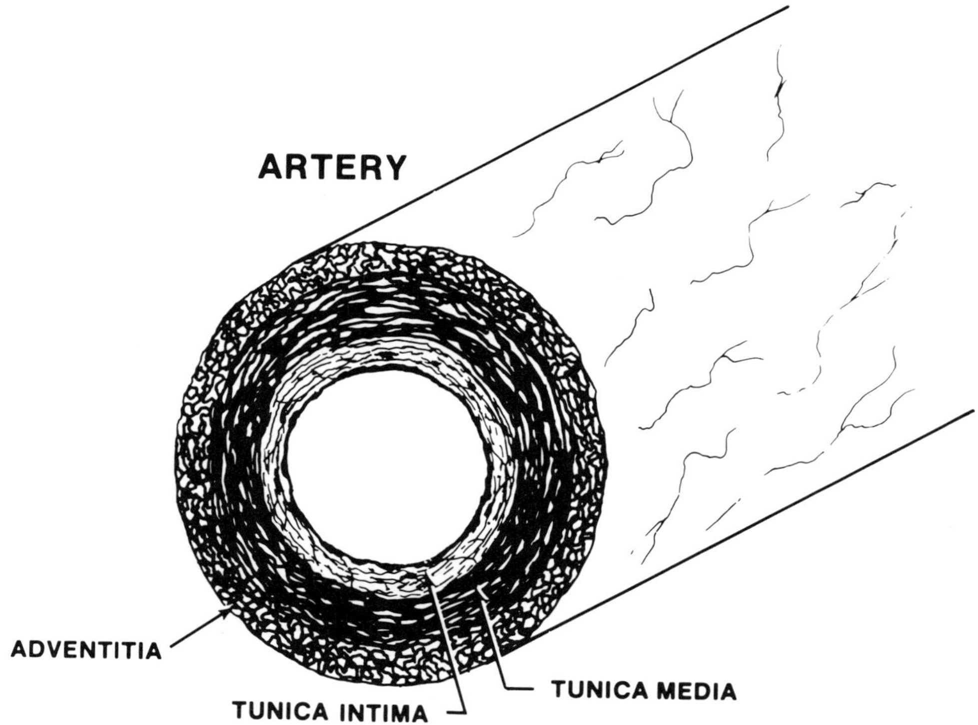

Figure 7.12

circuit. If arteriosclerotic plaque is present on the intimal surface of the artery, this plaque can be swept away by this jetting effect (Figure 7.13). This is particularly dangerous if the aorta is the site of arterial cannulation. The plaque can result in an embolus to the brain—a stroke. Arterial embolization can result in organ dysfunction or death.

When extensive arteriosclerotic plaque is present, just the event of blood reentry into the artery can cause pieces of plaque to break off and cause embolization.

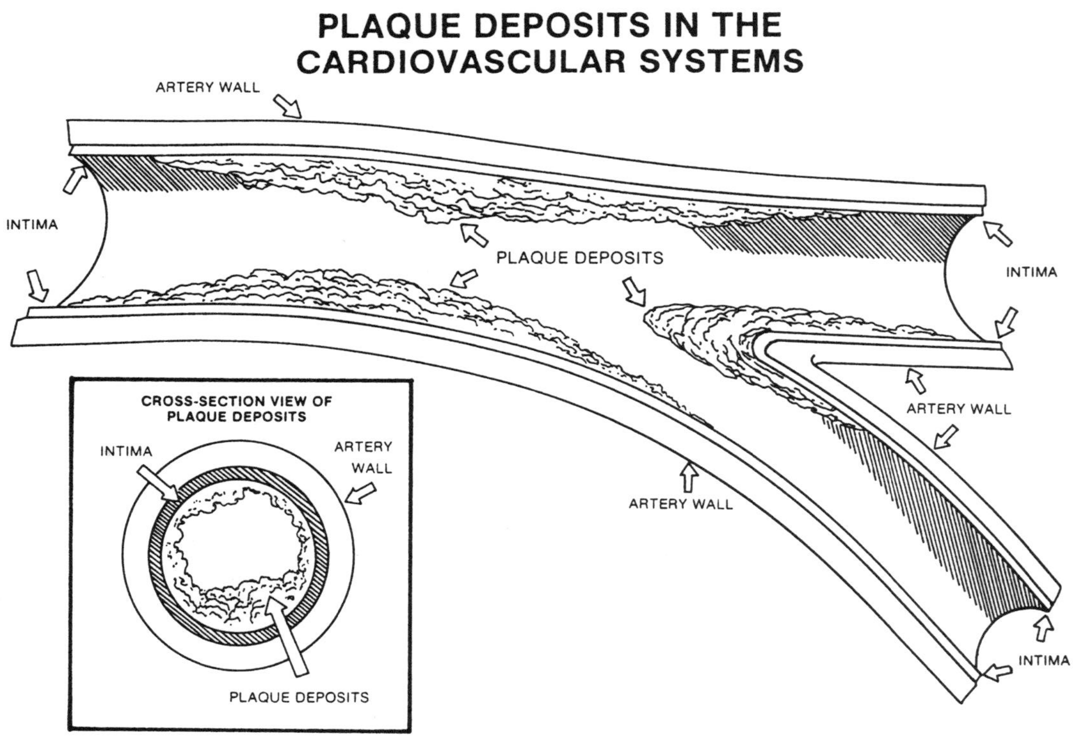

Figure 7.13 Plaque deposits on the intimal surface may be swept away, causing arterial embolization.

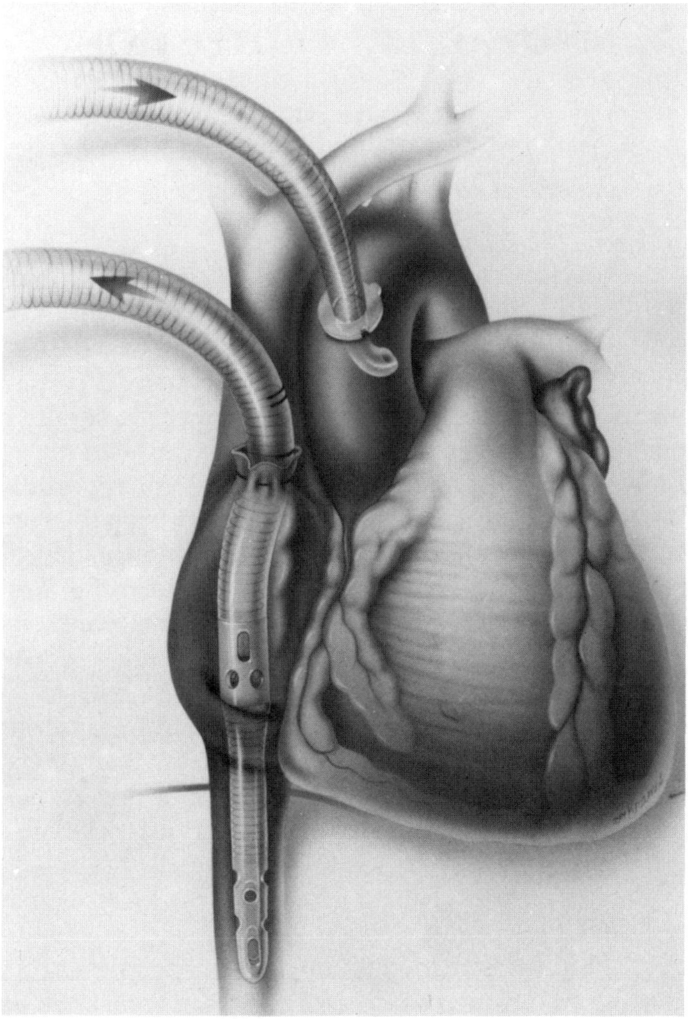

Figure 7.14 Cannulation of the heart during open-heart surgery. Dual stage venous cannulation and aortic arch cannulation of the aorta. (Courtesy of Research Medical, Inc., Salt Lake City, Utah.)

MYOCARDIAL PROTECTION

Chapter Eight

Protection of the Heart

The heart is composed of richly-vascularized muscle layers. It is the most mechanically active organ in the body, and it performs an enormous amount of work as it pumps blood throughout the circulatory system. Because of its work demands, the heart uses an immense quantity of oxygen. Oxygen-rich blood is supplied to the heart muscle by the heart's own arterial system—the coronary arteries (Figure 8.1). "Coronary" is a word derived from the Latin which means "to crown." Both coronary arteries, left and right, originate immediately above (distal to) the aortic valve. The left coronary divides into two main branches—the circumflex and the left anterior descending coronary arteries.

Because of its heavy work load and high oxygen requirements, the muscle mass of the heart can tolerate very little ischemia (reduction in blood supply to an area because of obstruction or constriction of the coronary arteries). When the blood supply is restricted to even a small area of heart muscle, a number of changes take place which decrease the heart's ability to pump blood.

Partial obstruction in the coronary arteries is most often caused by atherosclerosis, a disease in which plaques build up in the lumen of the coronary arteries, thus decreasing the amount of blood flow to an area of myocardium. As the disease progresses, the resulting ischemia of the myocardium may produce chest pain called "angina." Sometimes small branches of the coronaries become totally obstructed by plaque or by an embolus formed as a result of the plaque (Figure 8.2). When this occurs, the heart may develop severe rhythm disturbances, and the oxygen-deprived heart mus-

CORONARY ARTERIES

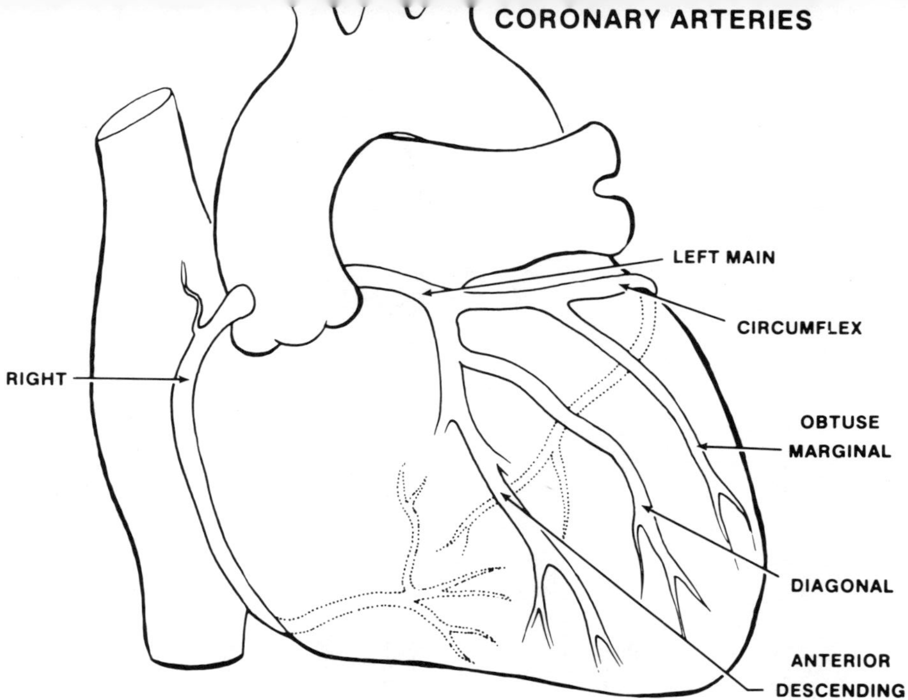

Figure 8.1

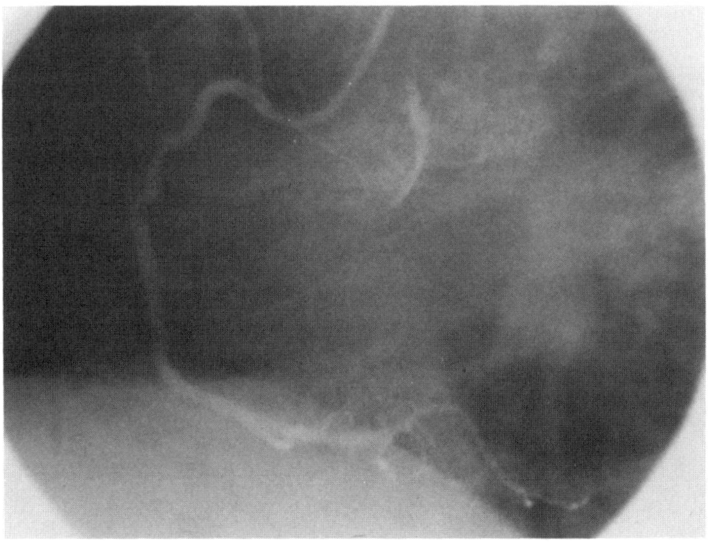

Figure 8.2 Radiopaque contrast medium is injected into the coronary arteries during cardiac catheterization to determine the degree of obstruction that has taken place during the athersclerotic disease process. The amount of obstruction is usually expressed as a percentage (e.g., the vessel is 90% obstructed). (Courtesy of E. Lawrence Ganter, M.D. (retired), Phoenix, Arizona.)

cle tissue dependent upon that artery will die. If total obstruction occurs in a main coronary artery or in a major branch, thus affecting a large area of myocardium, the heart will be unable to pump, and the individual will die.

During open heart surgery, the myocardial tissue must tolerate another kind of ischemia. Because the heart must be opened and motionless to accomplish the surgical correction, a variety of techniques have been employed to achieve a motionless heart while the patient's circulation is maintained to the rest of the body by a heart-lung machine (Figure 8.3). One such technique is to clamp off the aorta above (distal to) the point where the coronary arteries branch off, thereby preventing any blood to flow to the heart muscle by way of the coronaries. This technique, called "aortic cross-clamping," is performed in one of two ways. Either cross-clamping is performed intermittently (so that blood is allowed to flow through the coronaries for a period of time, followed by an ischemic period), or it is performed for the duration of the surgical procedure. Aortic cross-clamping has been performed for periods up to several hours. However, there are no known "safe" time parameters for cross-clamping. At the present time, there are better means of achieving a motionless heart.

Another technique used to allow a motionless heart, yet prevent total ischemia to the myocardium, is coronary perfusion (Figure 8.4). The aorta is cross-clamped as described before, but the coronary arteries are either cannulated individually, or the aorta is cannulated between the aortic valve and a cross-clamp. Oxygenated blood is pumped from an outlet in the artificial lung portion of the heart-lung machine directly into the coronary arterial system. Frequently, this blood is cooled with a separate heat exchanger so that it is cooler than the blood which perfuses the rest of the body, thus reducing the heart's oxygen consumption rate. This technique affords more protection to the stilled heart muscle than does cross-clamping alone. However, coronary perfusion is presently considered to be an "outmoded" technique.

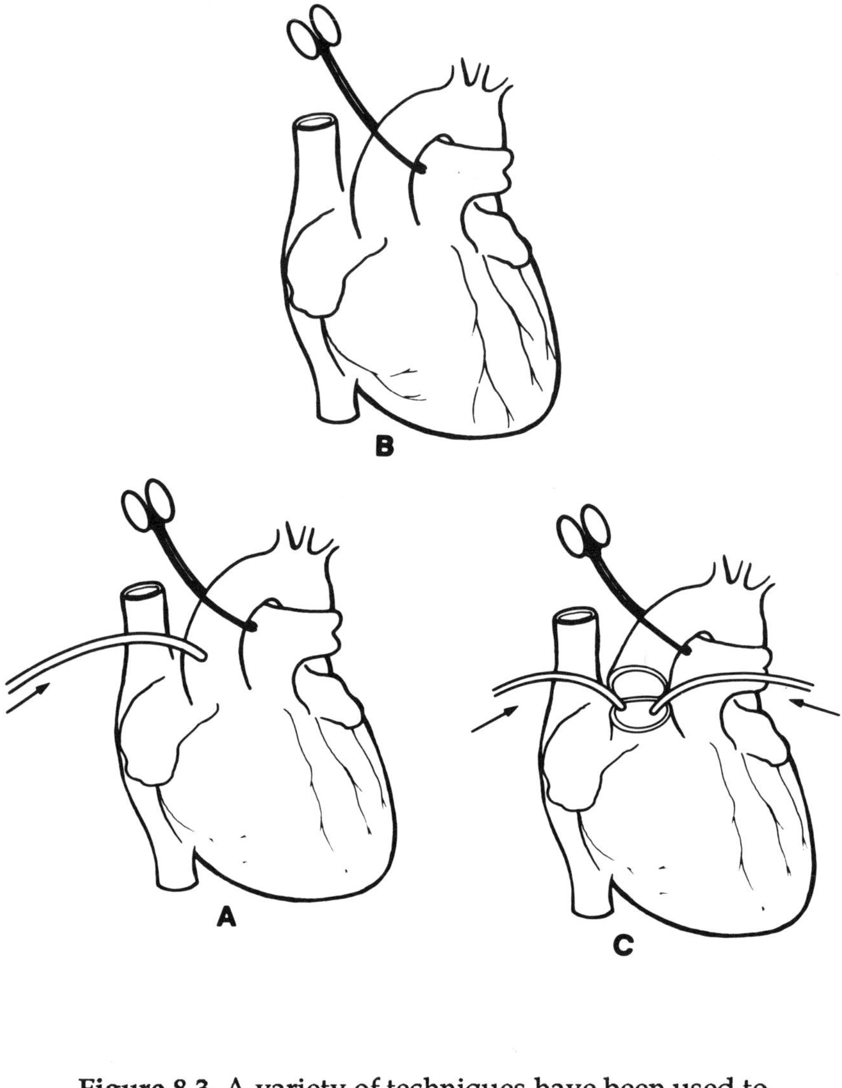

Figure 8.3 A variety of techniques have been used to achieve a motionless heart while the patient's circulation is maintained to the rest of the body by a heart-lung machine. (**A**) Cardioplegia solution is infused into the root of the aorta. (**B**) The aorta is cross-clamped, depriving the heart of blood. (**C**) The aorta is opened and the left and right coronary arteries are cannulated individually to deliver cardioplegia solution.

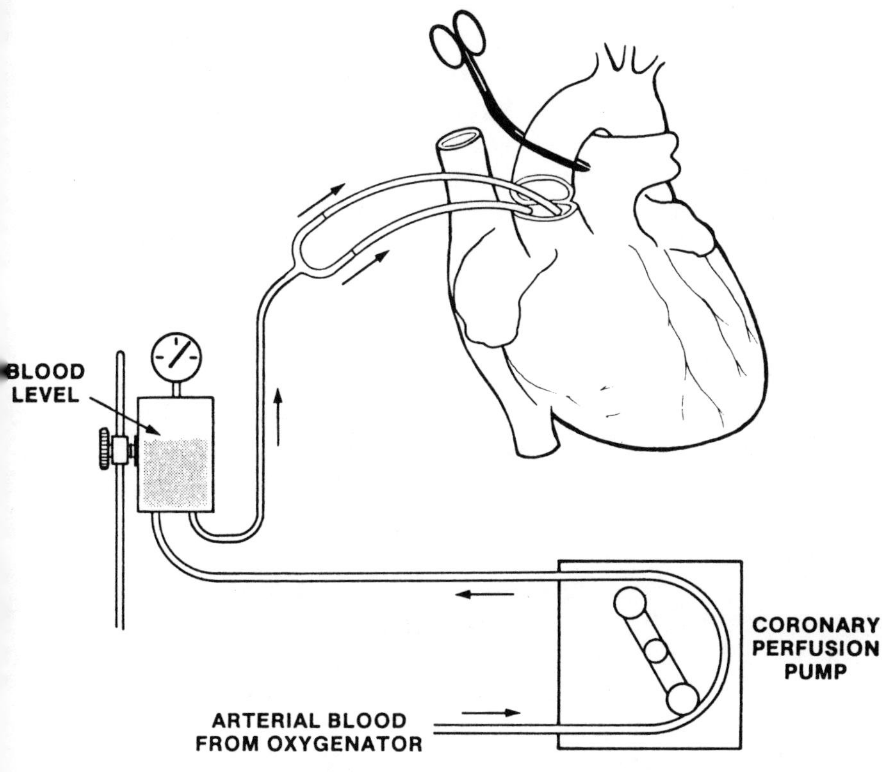

Figure 8.4 During coronary perfusion, a portion of the oxygenated blood is removed from the artificial lung and infused under pressure to the coronary arteries by a blood pump.

A more popular technique used to protect the ischemic myocardium involves the use of induced hypothermic cardioplegia. The technique involves the infusion of a cardioplegic solution into the coronary arteries at a low temperature. The chemical composition of the solution is varied; each cardiovascular surgical team has its own "recipe." However, the one chemical in common to all cardioplegic solutions is potassium. When infused, potassium causes an immediate arrest of the heart, and the low temperature immediately begins to reduce the heart's oxygen consumption rate. The immediate stoppage and rapid cooling of the myocardium seems to offer the maximum protection available at this time.

There are two kinds of cardioplegic methods: blood cardioplegia (Figure 8.5) and crystalloid cardioplegia (Figure 8.7). Blood cardioplegia is a solution which has been mixed with oxygenated blood from the extracorporeal circuit. A crystalloid cardioplegic solution is a noncellular solution that has a base of either normal saline or a balanced electrolyte (Figure 8.9).

The heart is commonly protected during open heart surgery for about an hour. Bayless, *et al*, has reported experimental myocardial protection using dog hearts for as long as 24 hours. Although there is a considerable amount of information available concerning what should constitute adequate myocardial protection, there are still no hard and fast rules about what constitutes a "safe period of ischemia." The only consensus is that myocardial ischemia should be maintained for as brief a period as possible.

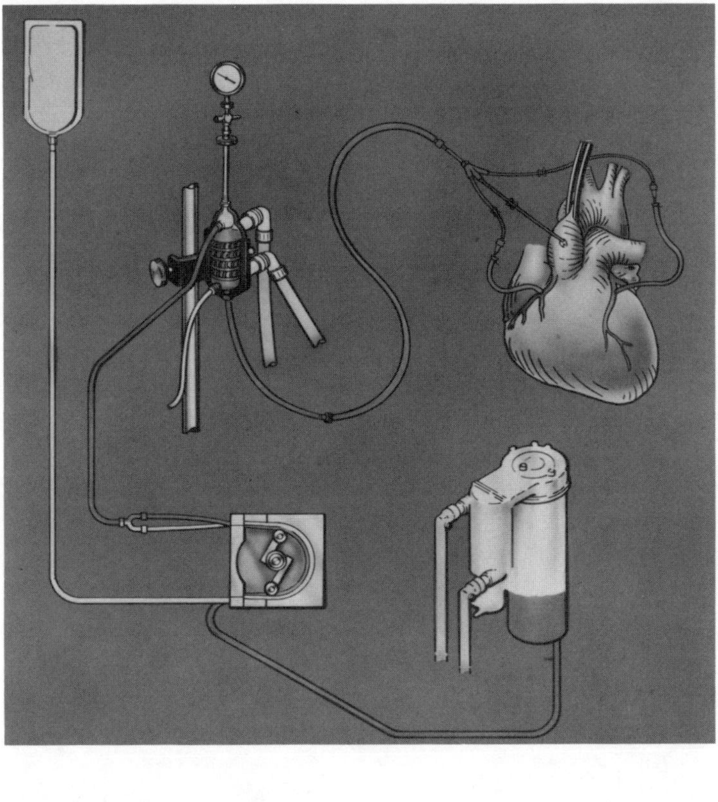

Figure 8.5 During the infusion of blood cardioplegia, a portion of the blood is removed from the artificial lung, mixed with a cardioplegia solution, cooled, and infused under pressure into the coronary arteries. (Courtesy of Shiley Laboratories, Santa Ana, California.)

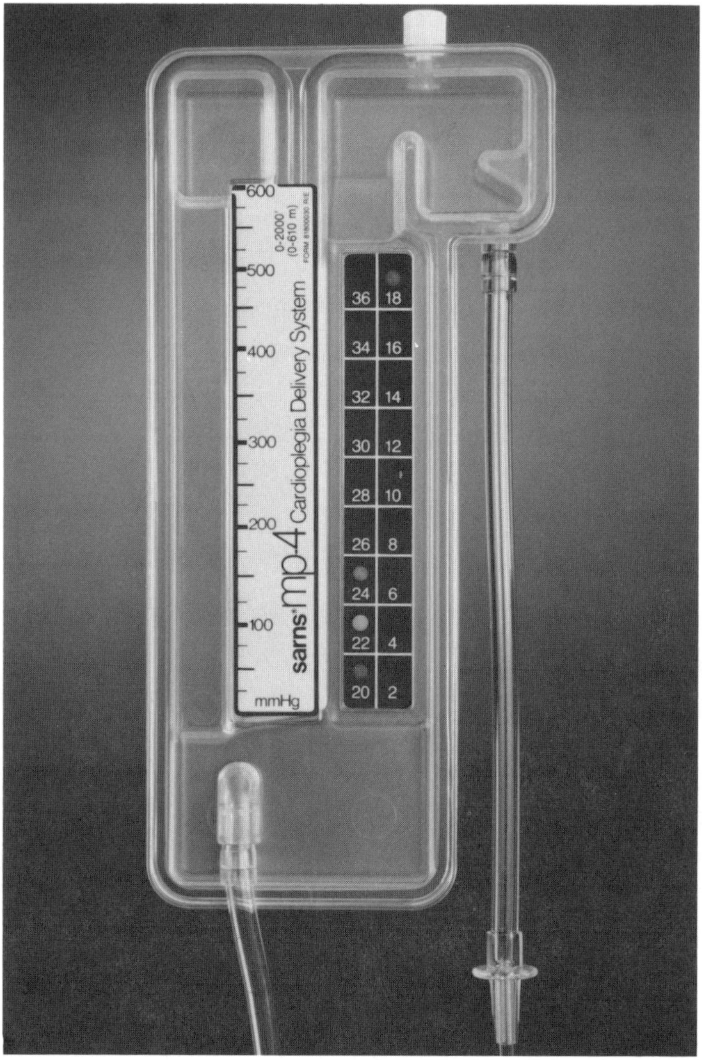

Figure 8.6 A blood cardioplegia set that has a built-in blood pressure monitoring module. (Courtesy of Sarns, 3M Healthcare, Ann Arbor, Michigan.)

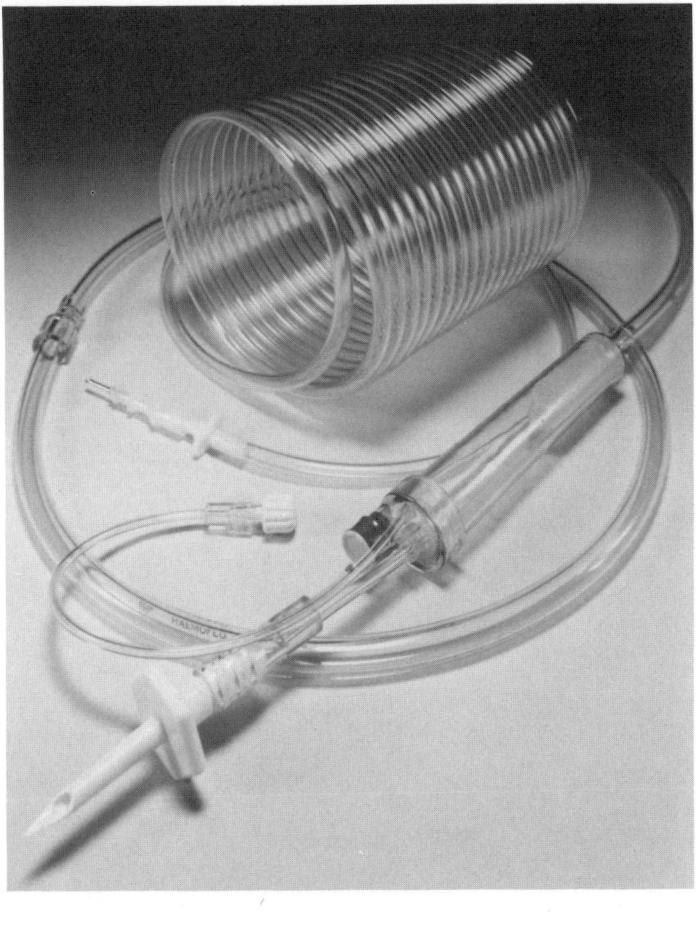

Figure 8.7 A number of cardioplegia infusion sets are commercially available. (Courtesy of Norton-Texas Medical Products, Houston, Texas.)

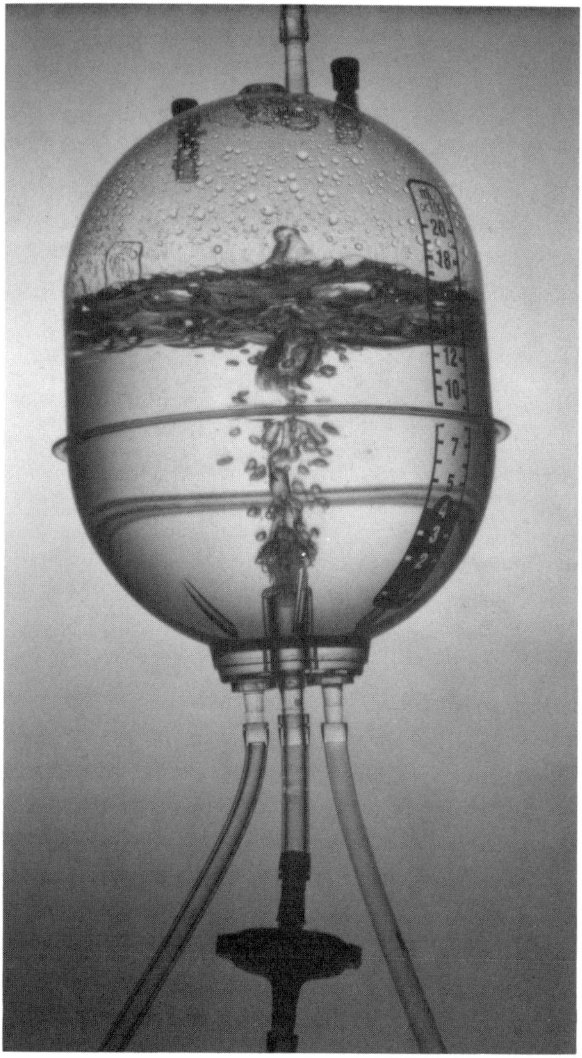

Figure 8.8 This cardioplegia (crystalloid) administration system provides a method to oxygenate the crystalloid cardioplegia solution. (Courtesy of Baxter Healthcare Corporation, Bentley Laboratories Division, Irvine, California.)

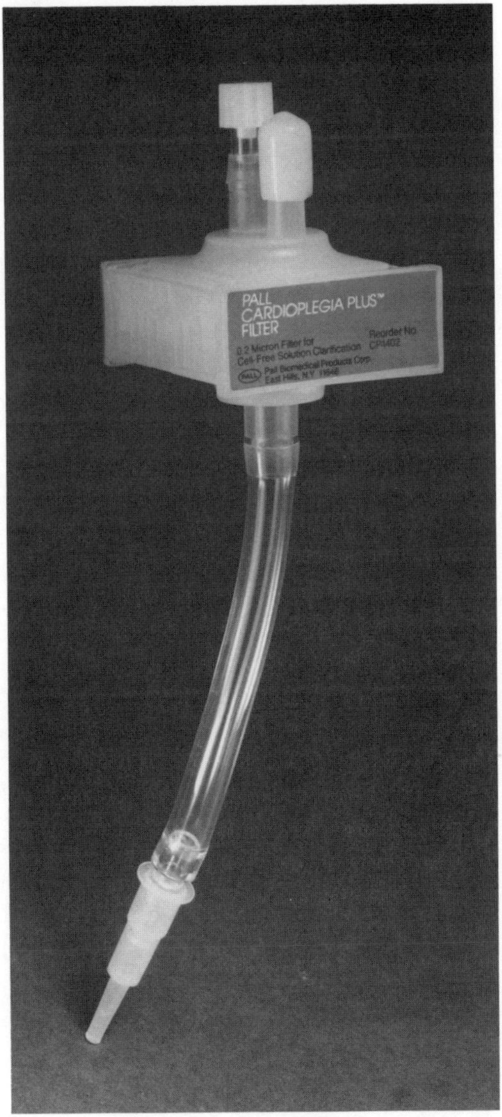

Figure 8.9 Some surgical teams filter the cardioplegia solution. (Courtesy of Pall Biomedical Corporation, Glen Cove, New York.)

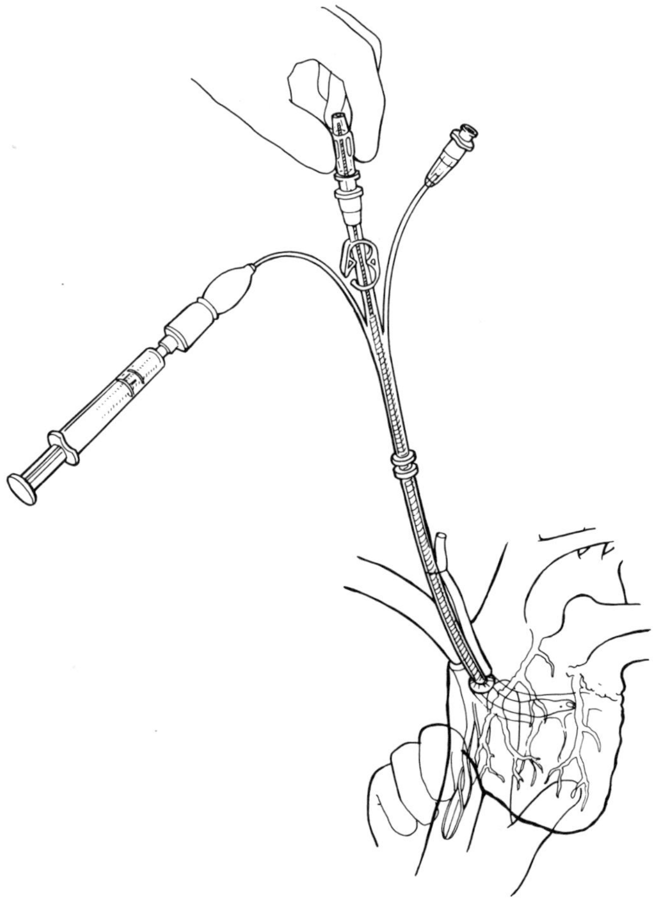

Figure 8.10 A cannula is placed in the coronary sinus in order to infuse cardioplegia retrograde to the coronary arteries. This process achieves hypothermic cardioplegia. (Courtesy of D.L.B., Inc., Grand Rapids, Michigan.)

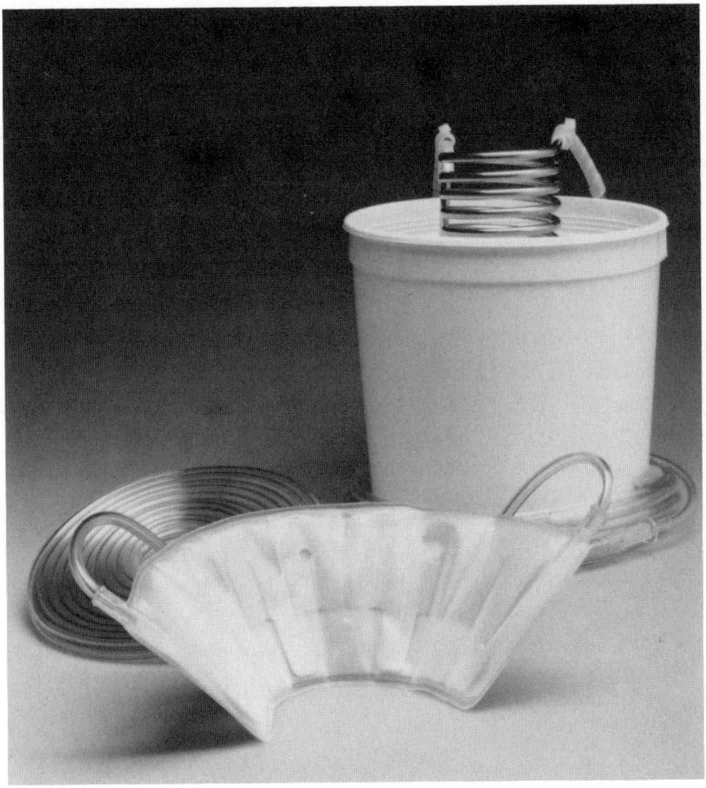

Figure 8.11 This cooling jacket is placed around the heart during open heart surgery. "Ice water" is circulated through the Cardiac Cooling Jacket to keep the heart cold. (Courtesy of Medtronic Blood Systems, Inc., Anaheim, California.)

HEMODYNAMIC CONSIDERATIONS

CHAPTER NINE

Blood Flow Rate

A blood flow rate during cardiopulmonary bypass should be as low as will effectively meet the metabolic needs of the patient. One reason is that blood trauma occurs in direct proportion to the total amount of blood flow through the extracorporeal apparatus. A second reason is that the operative procedure can be performed more expeditiously if large amounts of blood do not flood the operative site and obstruct the surgeon's view. Too, a slower heart lung machine operating speed is generally a safer speed to handle the blood. Bubble-type oxygenators are systems that have open blood reservoir levels. A minimum safe operating level has been defined by some to be a level that at a specified blood flow rate allows the perfusionist a 20 second reaction time. For example, if the specified blood flow rate is 4,500 ml/min and the oxygenator blood level is 1,500 ml, then it would take 20 seconds to drain the oxygenator.

At times, a lower cardiac output during cardiopulmonary bypass may be desireable to prevent excessive collateral circulation of blood through the heart when it is in a state of cardioplegic hypothermia. Preventing excessive collateral circulation to the coronaries not only prevents the heart from rewarming, it also prevents the heart from becoming perfused with oxygenated blood.

Total body hypothermia can allow a moderate reduction in blood flow rate by reducing the oxygen requirements of the patient. On some occasions, blood flow rates must be drastically slowed in order to carry out a proper surgical correction. At times, the perfusion can be stopped altogether for a short period of time with good results.

Ideal perfusion is not achievable because of the

limitation of less than perfect equipment and because of the demands of the operation itself. The way in which the heart-lung machine is operated is drastically influenced by the needs of the surgeon and by the condition of the patient.

Peripheral Vascular Resistance

Peripheral (systemic) vascular resistance is the opposing force offered to total blood flow. Various mathematical expressions have been devised with units quantified that meet the user's needs. Systemic vascular resistance is defined according to the General Blood Flow Equation:

$$\mathbf{SVR} = \frac{Pa\text{-}Pv}{Q} \times \frac{1}{n}$$

where Pa represents the mean arterial pressure, Pv represents the mean venous pressure, Q represents the cardiac output, and n represents the viscosity of the blood (Figure 9.1). Direct applications of this formula must be approached with caution since the blood is a non-newtonian fluid, and the body's circuit is a complex arrangement of distensible tubes. Also, blood viscosity is not a constant; it changes during the blood's transit through the circulatory system. For example, erythrocytes travel through the capillary system in single file, resulting in high frictional resistance (high viscosity) (Figure 9.2). Nevertheless, when used with caution, this expression of systemic vascular resistance is a valid and useful tool.

Changes in systemic vascular resistance become especially evident during total cardiopulmonary bypass. Cardiac output can be controlled at a constant rate. Observations can be made concerning what pressure will result from a given blood flow. A mean arterial pressure of between 60-80 mm Hg is considered to be unacceptable during a normothermic perfusion. Pressures as low as 50 mm Hg are acceptable during a hypothermic perfusion.

Low mean arterial pressures changes are often encountered during the first few minutes of cardiopulmonary bypass. It has been shown that this initial hypotension is due, in part, to a decrease in blood viscosity as a result of hemo-

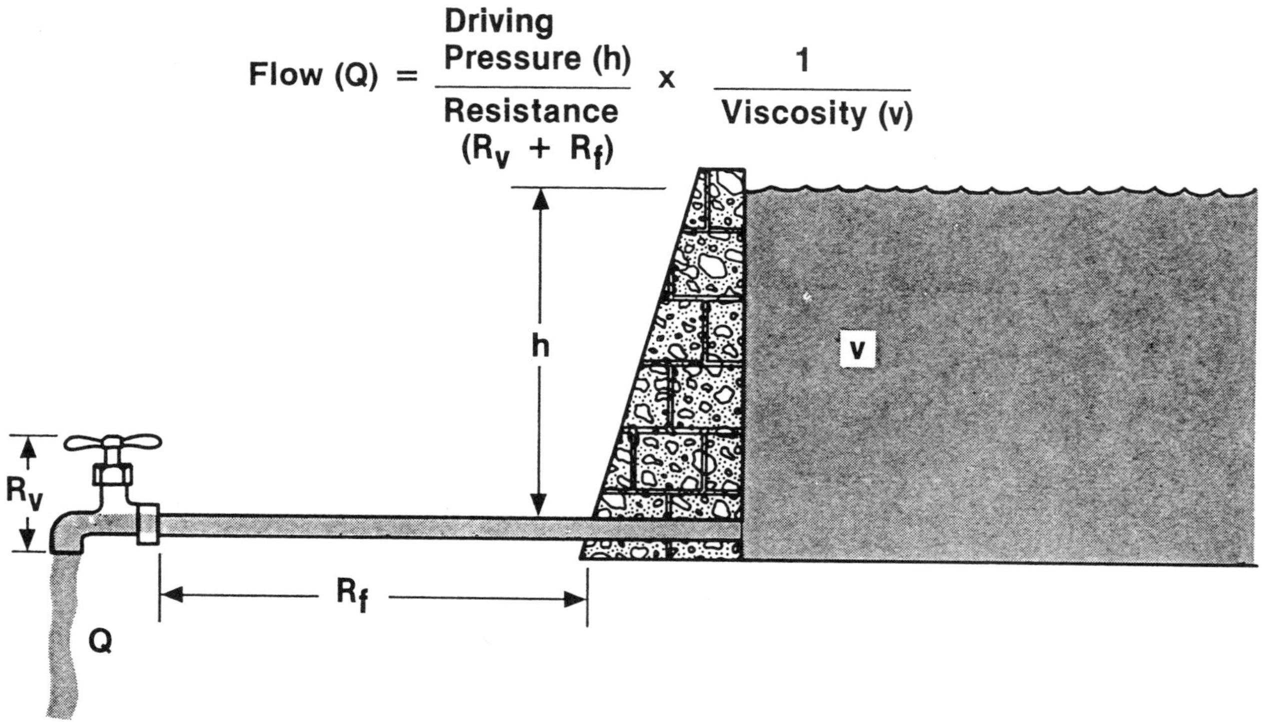

Figure 9.1 General Blood Flow Formula for calculating peripheral vascular resistance.

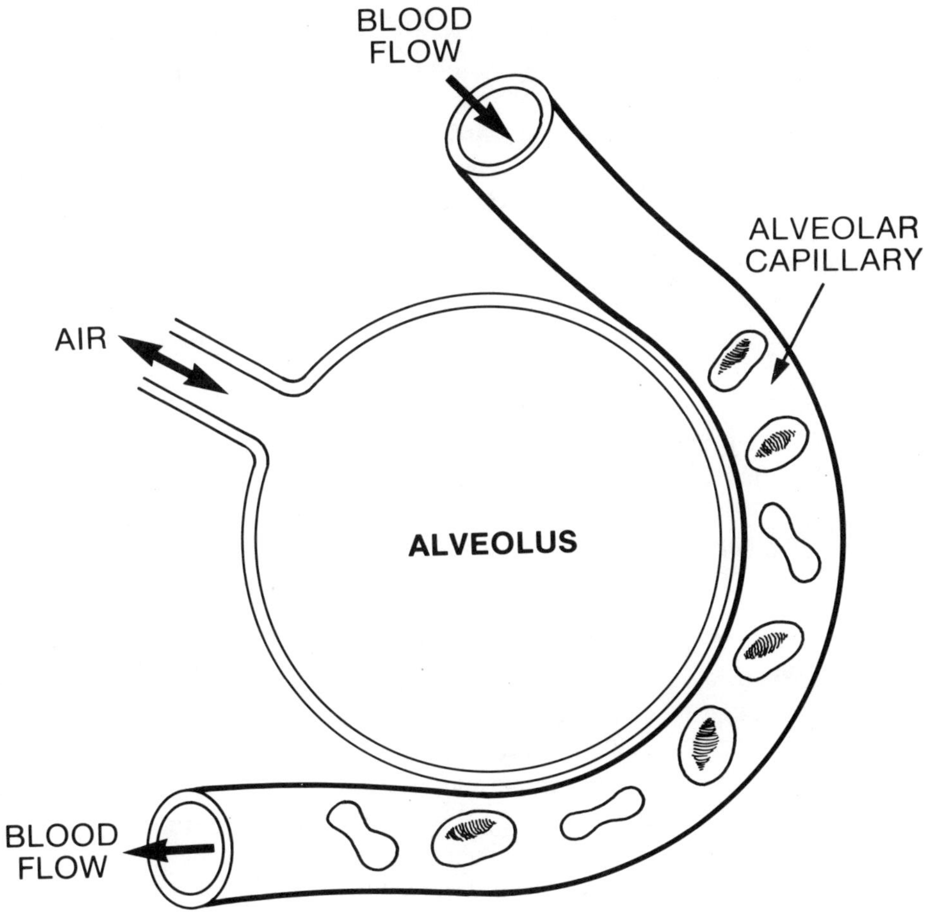

Figure 9.2 In much of the capillary system, erythrocytes must travel in single file.

dilution.

When initial hypotension is encountered, a temporary increase in total blood flow rate can usually be corrected by the perfusionist. Occasionally, vasopressor drugs are needed in small doses. Neo-synephrine is often the drug of choice. However, the use of any pressor agent during cardiopulmonary bypass should be avoided if possible.

It has been well-documented that total systemic vascular resistance increases with time during cardiopulmonary bypass. Excessively high blood pressure is not desireable. Increased pressures can contribute to tissue edema, excessive diuresis, and loss of serum electrolytes.

When preparing to "wean" a patient from cardiopulmonary bypass, the biochemical and hemodynamic parameters should be optimal in order for the patient to resume normal circulation. Optimum hemodynamic parameters are especially important if the patient's heart has less than ideal function. Low output failure or cardiac arrhythmias can seriously jeopardize the weaning of a patient from the extracorporeal apparatus.

A mathematical expression of systemic vascular resistance is a very useful tool to communicate the hemodynamic status of the patient to others in the surgical team. The administration of drugs which are capable of keeping the patient's systemic vascular resistance at its best level is not commonly administered by the perfusionist, but rather by the anesthesiologist. Excellent communication by all members of the surgical team is imperative at the critical time when a patient's heart is not strong enough to be weaned from the heart-lung machine.

It is not uncommon for an inexperienced perfusionist to attempt to maintain an adequate mean arterial blood pressure by decreasing the systemic blood flow when faced with increased systemic vascular resistance. However, this technique places an increased workload on the patient's heart by increasing the afterload on the heart. If the patient's heart is functioning poorly, it may have a difficult time to maintain an adequate cardiac output.

Likewise, faced with the patient's decreased systemic vascular resistance, the inexperienced perfusionist may drastically increase the total blood flow to compensate for the corresponding decrease in mean arterial pressure. When weaning this kind of patient from cardiopulmonary bypass, even if the patient has a left ventricle that is functioning well, the patient's cardiac output will not be able to maintain an adequate arterial pressure.

[A more detailed discussion of myocardial function and "weaning" from cardiopulmonary bypass may be found in Chapter Eleven.]

FLUID REQUIREMENTS

CHAPTER TEN

Priming Fluids

"Priming of the heart-lung machine" is defined as the process of putting the machine in working order by filling the machine with liquid. The liquid fills the empty spaces and displaces the atmospheric gases that are present. This displacement is called "de-bubbling," and is usually accomplished by recirculation. During the priming and debubbling phase, the perfusionist has an opportunity to check the machine for proper function.

During the early days of open heart surgery, heart-lung machines were primed with whole donor-blood. Many of these early machines had large priming volumes which required from 8 to 10 units (500 ml/unit) of donor blood to fill the machine to a safe operating level (Figure 10.1). Donor blood was drawn fresh, that is, within 24 hours of use and was anticoagulated with sodium heparin. Donor blood procurement problems were immense—as were the costs. These machines could not be operated in an emergency because of their large priming volumes. Although the blood was cross-matched against the patient's own blood, minor blood incompatibilities were an ever present problem because of the large number of donors required. These incompatibilities caused what was then called "the blood pool syndrome." Not only was the incidence of blood transfusion reactions a problem, but there was also a high incidence of diseases, such as hepatitis, that were transmitted by donor blood transfusion.

During the next historical phase in the progress of extracorporeal circulation, partial hemodilution was used extensively. Pump oxygenator systems were primed in part with glucose solutions, such as 5% dextrose in water. Although there was a decrease in the oxygen-carrying capacity

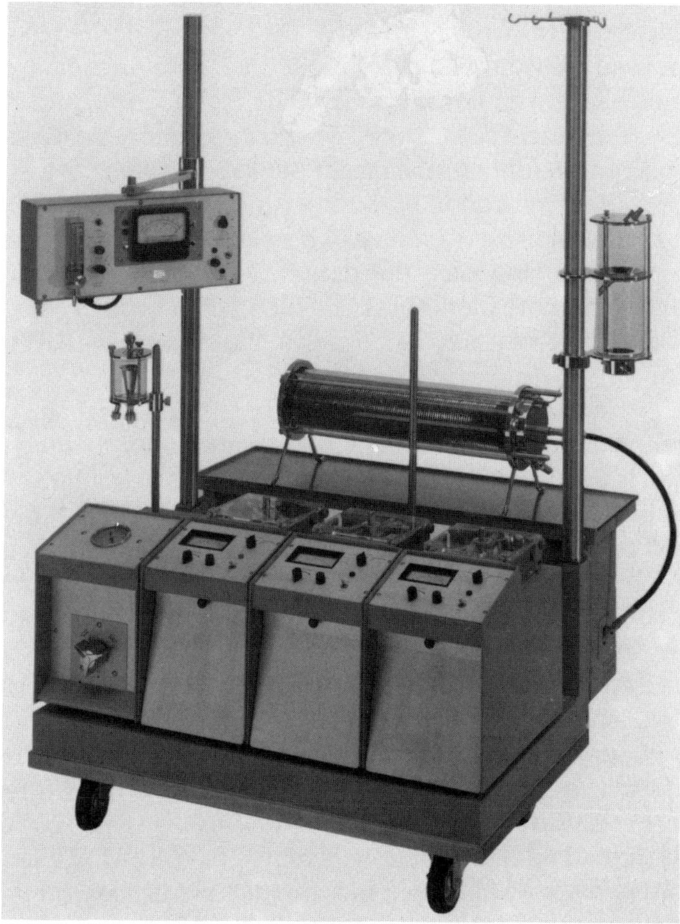

Figure 10.1 Many of the earlier models of heart-lung machines required large amounts of priming blood volume. (Courtesy of Sarns, 3M Healthcare, Ann Arbor, Michigan.)

of the blood, there was an improvement in capillary level circulation made by decreasing the viscosity of the circulating blood. When hemodilution was combined with hypothermia, there was a noticeable improvement in the micro circulation over that achieved with blood priming. As the blood temperature was lowered, the viscosity of the blood increased. It was then discovered that heparinization of donor blood was not necessary. The blood cells could be preserved in an Acid-Citrate-Phosphate solution, then used for priming volume. Problems still existed because of diseases transmitted by donor blood transfusion, but they were lessened because of the decreased volume of blood needed for priming. However, the donor blood's red cells were found to be more fragile in stored blood than in fresh blood. These cells were easily damaged by the extracorporeal circuit.

In the present phase of priming fluids, total hemodilution primes have evolved. This is not to say that some blood is not required in the prime, but such use is relatively rare in perfusing adult patients. Total hemodilution allows rapid deployment of the heart-lung machine in emergencies. Total hemodilution is also the most cost-effective way to prime a heart-lung machine. Many of the total hemodilution primes use a balanced electrolyte solution, such as Lactated Ringer's. This kind of prime is a noncellular, crystalloid solution. Occasionally, albumin or heta starch is added to some primes to increase their oncotic pressure (pressure caused by large molecules). This kind of additive may be used in a patient, for example, who has a small blood volume and who may be excessively hemodiluted. Sodium bicarbonate may be added to buffer the pH of the priming solution to a physiological level (Figure 10.3). Some primes contain glucose solution, Mannitol, and heparin. The formula or "recipe" used for pump priming is extremely varied from institution to institution. Packed red blood cells will sometimes be added to the priming solution if the mixed hematocrit (the resultant hematocrit of the blood when mixed with the pump prime) is predicted to be at a lower

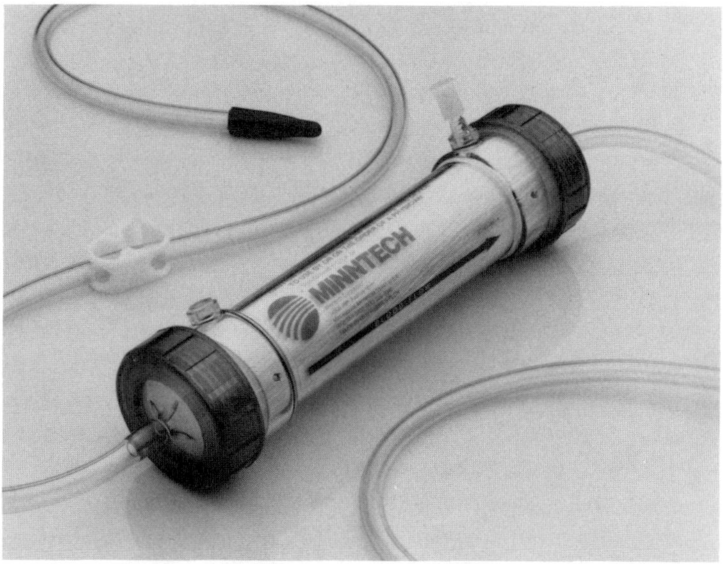

Figure 10.2 Hemoconcentration can be accomplished in an extracorporeal circuit by the use of a hemoconcentrator (a device that works like the kidney). (Courtesy of Minntech Corporation, Minneapolis, Minnesota.)

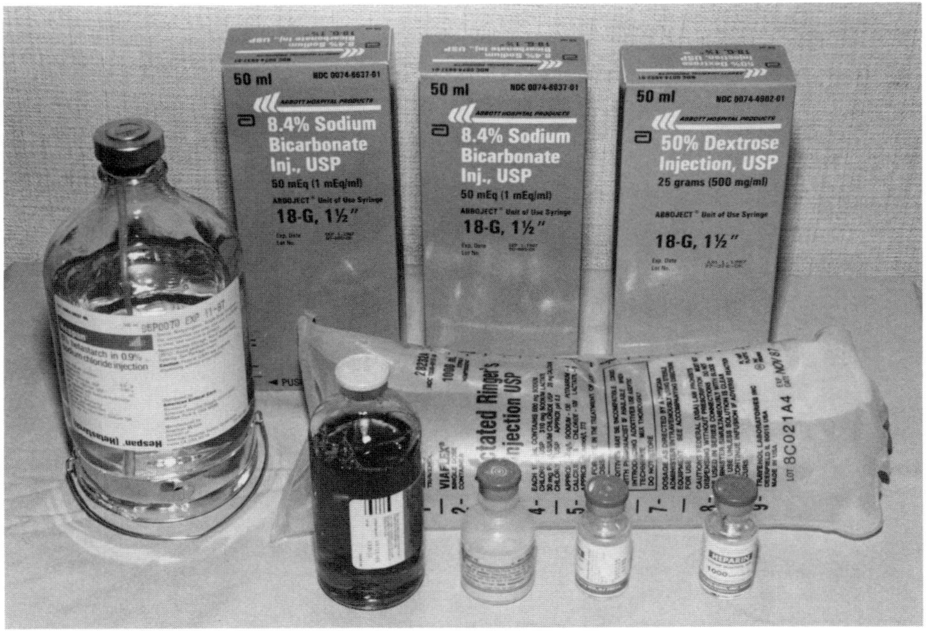

Figure 10.3 Many constituents can be added to the heart-lung machine for priming.

than desirable physiological level.

Blood Transfusion

It is in man's nature to seek rebirth or new life. Greek literature and other ancient writings contain many references to replacing the blood of aging heroes or patriarchs with "elixirs" to restore their youth and vigor. Ovid, a Roman poet who lived and wrote about the time of the birth of Christ, made mention of such a process in his *Metamorphoses*. In this work, Jason, the young hero, pleads with Medea, his lover, to restore the youth of his father, King Aeson.

> Medea took her unsheathed knife and cut the old man's throat, letting all of his old blood out of him. She filled his ancient veins with a rich elixir. Received it through his lips and wound, his beard and hair no longer white with age, turned quickly to their natural vigor, dark and lustrous; and his wasted form renewed, appeared in all the vigor of bright youth.[1]

Among the ancients, drinking blood was often recommended as a cure for diseases such as leprosy and epilepsy.

In the Book of Deuteronomy in the Old Testament of the *Holy Bible,* Moses cited The Ten Commandments and other laws of conduct to the people of Israel. One such law, found in the twelfth chapter, regulated the sacrificial use of meat and the eating of meat. While the law condoned ritual slaughter and eating meat of various kinds, it forbade "eating" (or drinking?) the blood of animals, from either sacrificial animals or from those killed for food. While some biblical scholars interpret this law simply as a dietary prohibition (other more primitive cultures in that part of the world did eat and drink blood), some religious groups have interpreted these biblical passages as prohibiting modern donor blood transfusions.

There are many other early references and allusions

to the ingestion and transfusion of blood, but little scientific attention was paid to blood transfusion until the seventeenth century. The event that stimulated scientific interest was the description of the circulation of blood by William Harvey, as mentioned in the first chapter of this book. During that century, there were several people who claimed that they were the first to transfuse blood. A recluse, one Frances Potter, documented the idea of transfusion in the writings of a contemporary in 1639. He designed quills and tubes for the procedure, but when he attempted it on a chicken ten years later, the experiment failed.[2]

In 1656, Sir Christopher Wren, the English architect famed for his designs of cathedrals and other major structures, first proposed administering medications to dogs intravenously by means of an animal bladder attached to quills. Other experimenters refined this idea by designing two small silver cannulae connected to a small leather bag.[3]

A contemporary of Wren, an English physician by the name of Richard Lower, demonstrated a blood transfusion between two dogs, and seems to be the first person to have defined the appropriateness of transfusion in cases of severe hemorrhage. He was able to show that a dog could be bled almost to the point of death, then could recover by means of a transfusion. However, the famous diarist, Samuel Pepys, who recorded one of Lower's experiments in his diary, believed the procedure could be "...of mighty use to man's health, for the amendment of bad blood by borrowing from a better body."[4]

Other experiments followed in rapid succession, including those transfusing animal blood into humans. A young French physician, Jean Denis, who was a member of King Louis XIV's staff, is credited with performing the first successful animal-to-human transfusions in 1667. He transfused a boy whose illness was associated with extreme weakness (likely related to multiple bloodlettings), a 45 year old man (apparently for no clinical reason), the son of a foreign dignitary, and a hemiplegic woman. All of these transfusions were apparently successful. Denis preferred animal blood because it was less likely to "be rendered impure by passion or vice." However, Denis's further experiments created jealousy among other Parisian physicians, and their efforts to discredit him succeeded. The Faculty of Medicine of Paris decreed that transfusions were considered criminal acts in the City of Paris unless approved by the Faculty. The French Parliament followed with a law that forbade transfusions in the whole of France, and The Royal Society in London followed suit for England. The crowning blow was the banning of transfusions by the Pope, and the scientific community of the Western World lost interest in the procedure.[5]

It was not until 1900 that Landsteiner described the now universally-known ABO blood typing system. He found that blood can be categorized into four major types: O, A, B, and AB. Type O blood is the most common; Type AB is the least common. In 1937, Landsteiner and Weiner identified another factor, an antigen, involved with blood compatibility. They named this factor the "rhesus factor" (Rh) because the researchers used rhesus monkeys in the blood experiments. If the Rh factor is present in the blood, blood is identified as "Rh positive." If the factor is absent, the blood is termed "Rh negative."[6]

The first blood bank was established in Cook County, Illinois in 1937. But it was not until World War II that whole blood transfusions and blood plasma transfusions were used extensively, saving thousands of lives. These advances opened the way for more complex surgical procedures, including open heart surgery.

Today, there are more than 50 identifiable blood factors. Most of these antigen-antibody reactions involve clumping (agglutination) of the red cells.

Many diseases, such as malaria, hepatitis, and AIDS, can be transmitted by donor blood transfusion (Figure 10.4). Because of this risk and because of the complexity and expense of such transfusions, most open heart surgical teams try to minimize their use. It is to the credit of highly-skilled blood bank and clinical laboratory physicians and technicians throughout the world that donor blood transfusions may be used with relative safety.

Autotransfusion

The need for blood replacement has probably been obvious to humans from the time that blood loss was associated with death. Surely it must have occurred to primitive man that if lost blood could be returned to an exsanguinating person, life might be preserved. The return of that blood, the person's own blood, to the body is now common. Its modern names are "intraoperative autotransfusion" or "autologous blood transfusion." .

Historically, there were many attempts to use autotransfusion. In 1818, Dr. James Blundell was a lecturer at Guy's Hospital in London on the subject of midwifery. At this point in medical history, severe postpartum hemorrhage usually meant death to the new mother. However, Dr. Blundell autotransfused ten such patients. Five survived.

In 1885, Dr. John Duncan reported the use of intraoperative autotransfusion following an leg amputation. He collected three ounces of blood in a dish containing phosphate of soda as an anticoagulant. The collected blood was reinfused into a vein of the stump of the amputated limb. Duncan's successful amputation and application of autotransfusion led him to use the procedure in other cases. He was convinced that "...this little operation..." would save many lives.[7]

Sporadically, other uses of intraoperative autotransfusion were reported in the surgical literature. However, with the increased interest in donor transfusion in the early 1900's, interest in autotransfusion waned.

Dr. Richard Dyer pioneered a renewed interest in intraoperative autotransfusion in the late 1960s. Dr. Dyer's work was followed by that of Dr. Gerald Klebanoff, which lead to the development of the first commercial auto-transfusion apparatus, marketed by Bentley Laboratories of Santa Ana, California (Figure 10.5).

In more recent times, autotransfusion has been used

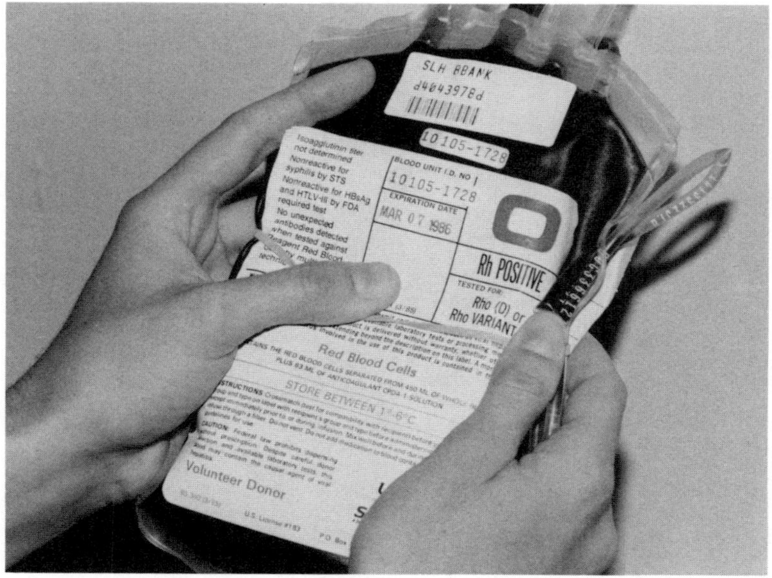

Figure 10.4 Donor blood is carefully screened for a number of diseases prior to perfusion. (Photo by William Jobe, Phoenix, Arizona.)

most often in cases involving severe hemorrhage. Surgeons are accustomed to see large quantities of blood suctioned from the operative wound, measured, and replaced with cross-matched donor blood. Indeed, donor blood still serves as the most common source for blood replacement. However, no one can dispute the facts. Donor blood transfusions do carry a certain amount of risk, and logic tells us that hypovolemic patients would be better off to receive identical blood (their own) (Figure 10.6). The time involved in obtaining and cross-matching whole blood or even in obtaining plasma may result in death if hemorrhaging is severe.[8]

There are other reasons for collecting and reinfusing the patient's own blood. In addition to compatibility, the temperature of autotransfused blood usually more closely approximates body temperature than refrigerated donor blood. Viable clotting factors exist in autotransfused blood that do not exist in stored donor blood. Intraoperative autotranfusion can overcome religious objections (such as those expressed by Jehovah's Witnesses) to donor blood. As donor blood becomes harder to get, especially in times of disaster and war, and in rural and remote areas, autotransfusion can often be used in lieu of scarce donor blood.

The processes involved with intraoperative blood autotransfusion are collection, anticoagulation, filtration, and reinfusion (Figure 10.7). There are problems associated with each process. For example, blood for autotransfusion is usually collected from the surgical cavity by active vacuum—just as it is used in the cardiotomy suction system of the heart lung machine. This kind of suction system causes a significant amount of blood trauma, a serious problem. Hemolysis of the red cells results in blood that has decreased oxygen-carrying capacity (anemia). Damage to the platelets and the plasma proteins can impair the clotting mechanism.

Anticoagulation is closely tied to the problems of collection. Autotransfused blood must not clot in the collection or reinfusion apparatus. The management of anticoagulation has been accomplished by the aid of three drugs: acid-citrate-dextrose (ACD), citrate-phosphate-dextrose

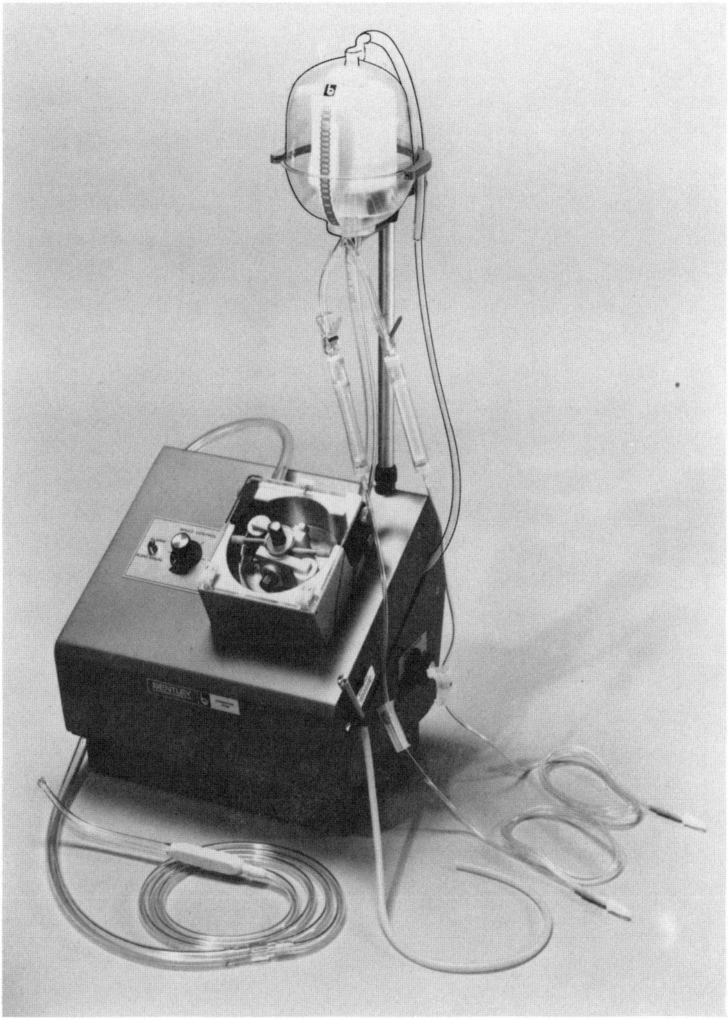

Figure 10.5 The Bentley intraoperative autotransfusion system was one of the first commercially-available autotransfusion devices. (Courtesy of Baxter Healthcare Corporation, Bentley Laboratories Division, Irvine, California.)

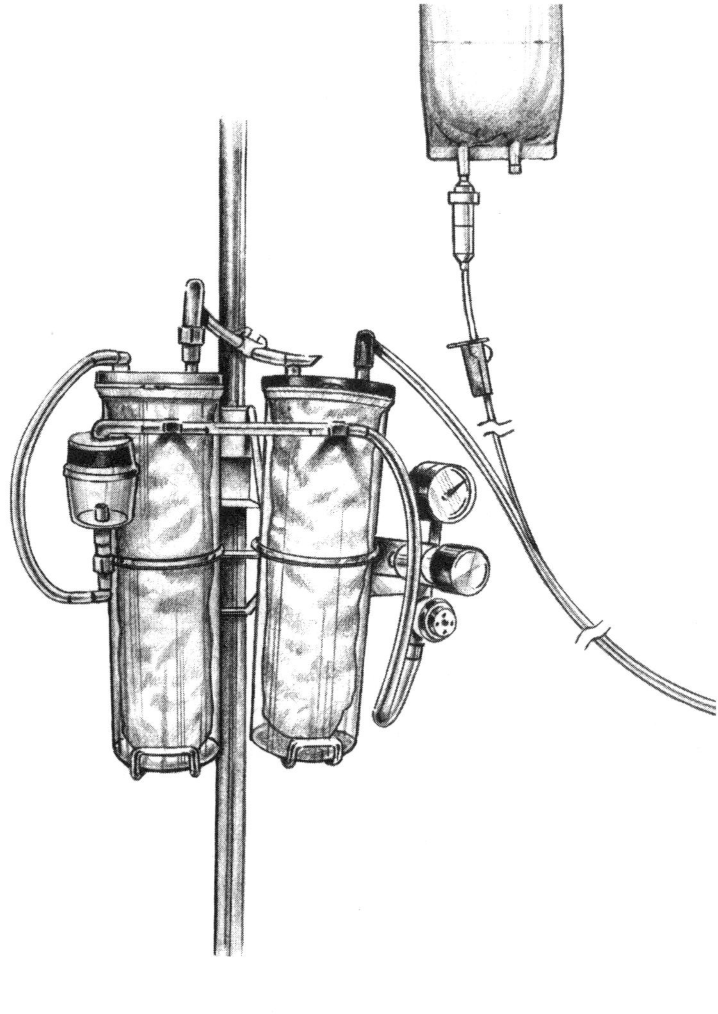

Figure 10.6 Many systems have been devised for the collection and reinfusion of patients' blood. (Courtesy of Sorenson Research Company, Inc., Salt Lake City, Utah.)

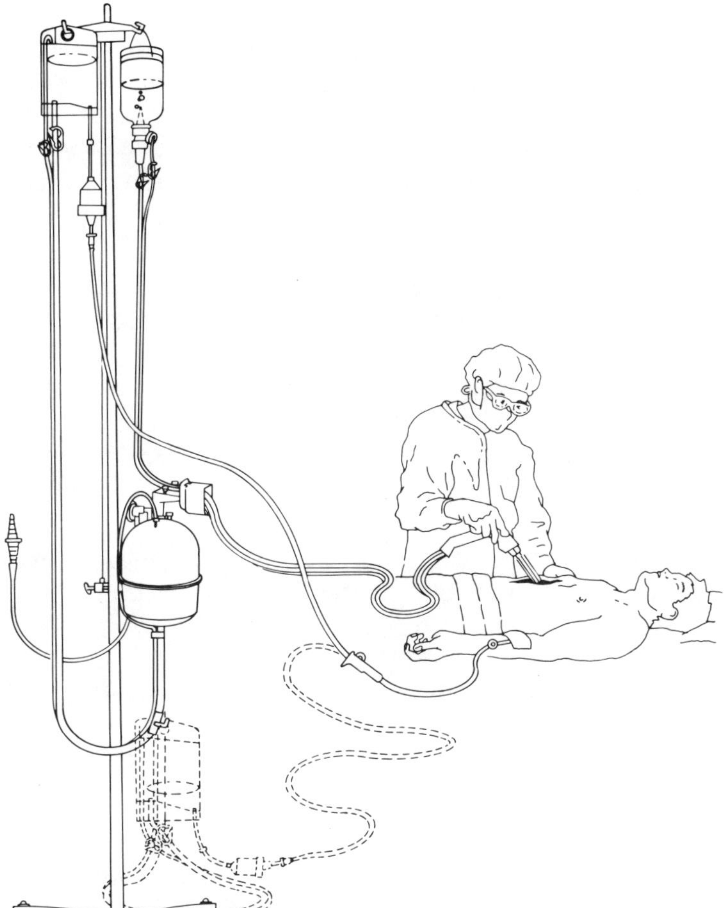

Figure 10.7 Collection-reinfusion system designed so that the anticoagulant is mixed at the suction tip. (Courtesy of Thoratec Laboratories Corporation, Berkeley, California.)

(CPD), and heparin. The choice of anticoagulant is debatable and depends on the kind of autotransfusion apparatus that is used.

Cellular debris, a result of blood trauma and micro-aggregates, can lead to clogging of the lung capillary beds, causing pulmonary hypertension (Figure 10.8). This kind of problem results because the autotransfused blood is infused into the venous system and is immediately circulated to the lungs for oxygenation. To reduce micro-aggregates, a micro-emboli filtration system is used prior to reinfusion, just as in the cardiotomy suction system.

The relatively small volume of blood that can be reinfused if the blood is infused through a very small intravenous needle can be a problem.

A bacterially-contaminated wound, such as one found in a penetrating injury to the intestines, contraindicates intraoperative autotransfusion. However, some experts feel that the use of this "contaminated" blood is better than no blood at all in a "life or death" emergency.

Several intraoperative autotransfusion systems are commercially available. Most of them involve the collection and filtration of the blood in a reservoir similar to the cardiotomy reservoir (Figure 10.9). Several of these systems collect the blood to be autotransfused, then separate the blood components by centrifugation. Red cells settle to the bottom of a "bowl," while the plasma rises and is removed from the top. The red cells can then be "washed" with saline and returned to the patient. The product of this system is a unit of "packed red cells." The washing process also eliminates all of the white cells, the platelets, and the viable plasma protein fraction from the blood. The packed red cells are used to increase the oxygen-carrying capacity of the patient's blood.

An additional benefit of intraoperative blood salvage is the peace-of-mind that patients can derive from knowing that they cannot receive contaminated blood (hepatitis, AIDS, etc.) by this method. In addition, patients receiving auto-transfused blood have the satisfaction of knowing

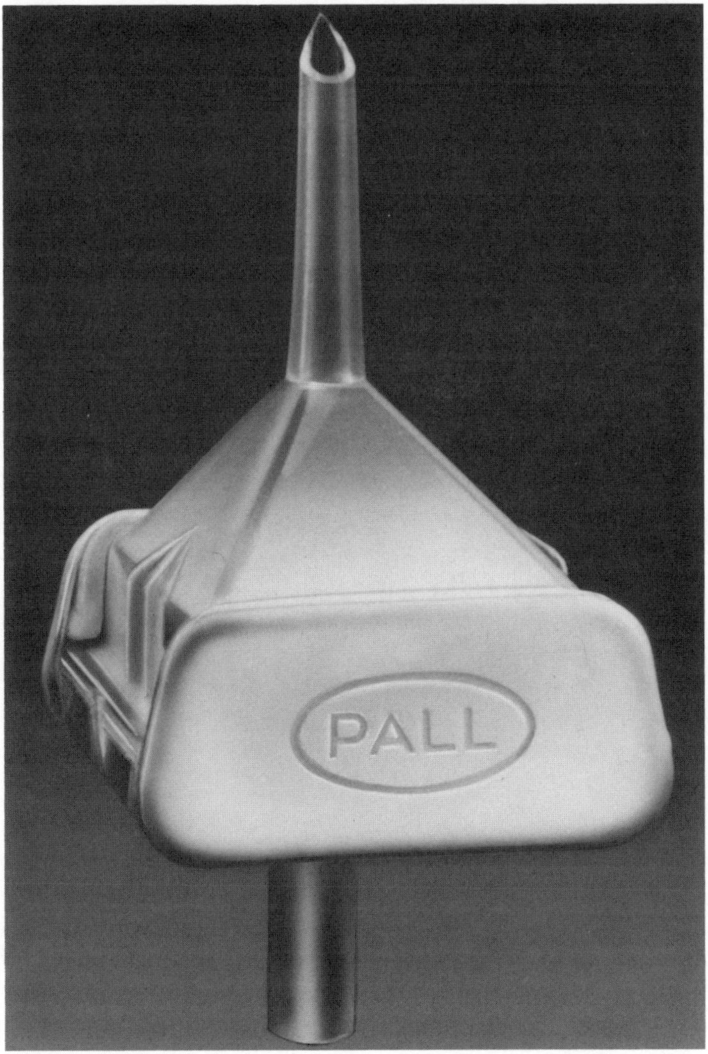

Figure 10.8 Cellular debris must be removed from the blood prior to infusion into the patient.

that they have conserved the precious supply of donor blood.

At the conclusion of cardiopulmonary bypass, some blood may remain in the extracorporeal circuit. This remaining blood has been diluted by the priming solution, but it can be hemoconcentrated by the use of centrifugation and returned to the patient. Another reason a washing process is necessary is to remove heparin. This avoids systemic anticoagulant effects that would be brought about by reinfusing "unwashed" blood.

It is also possible to hemoconcentrate by the use of ultra-filtration with an artificial kidney-type system. The ultra-filtration system retains the viable plasma fraction of the blood and removes the excess plasma water. It does not, however, remove the heparin. Still, both techniques are used successfully by open heart surgery teams.

It seems quite predictable that the use of intraoperative autotransfusion will increase in this technological and cost-conscious age. The process seems especially desirable when diseases such as AIDS and hepatitis may result in increased mortality for the patient who is donor transfused.

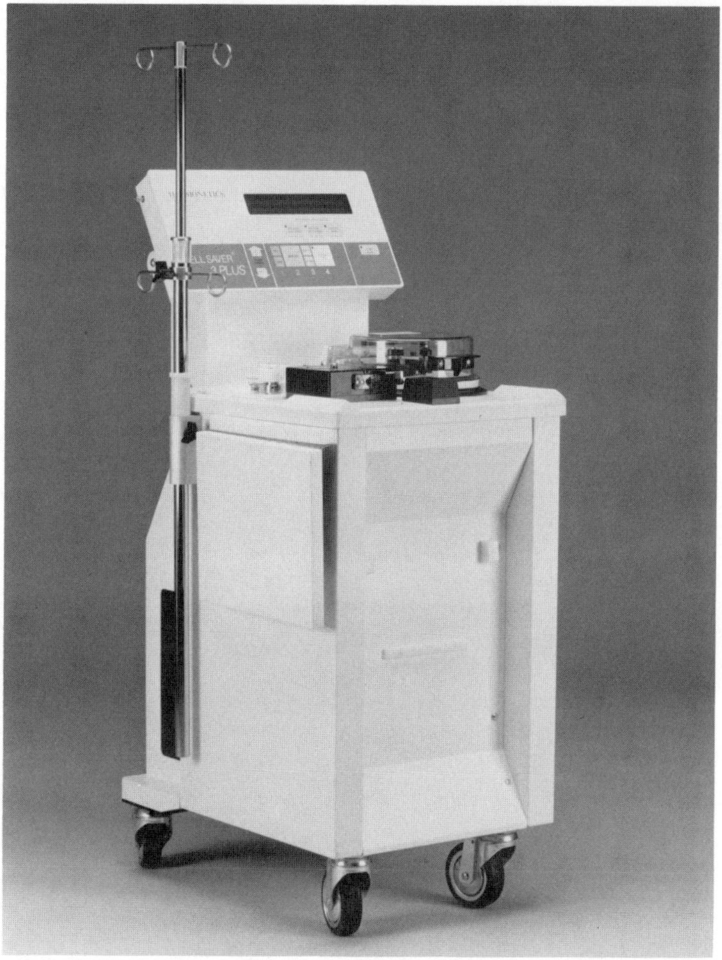

Figure 10.9 Autologous blood may be reinfused into the patient after centrifugation and washing of the red blood cells. (Courtesy of Baxter Healthcare Corporation, Bentley Laboratories Division, Irvine, California.)

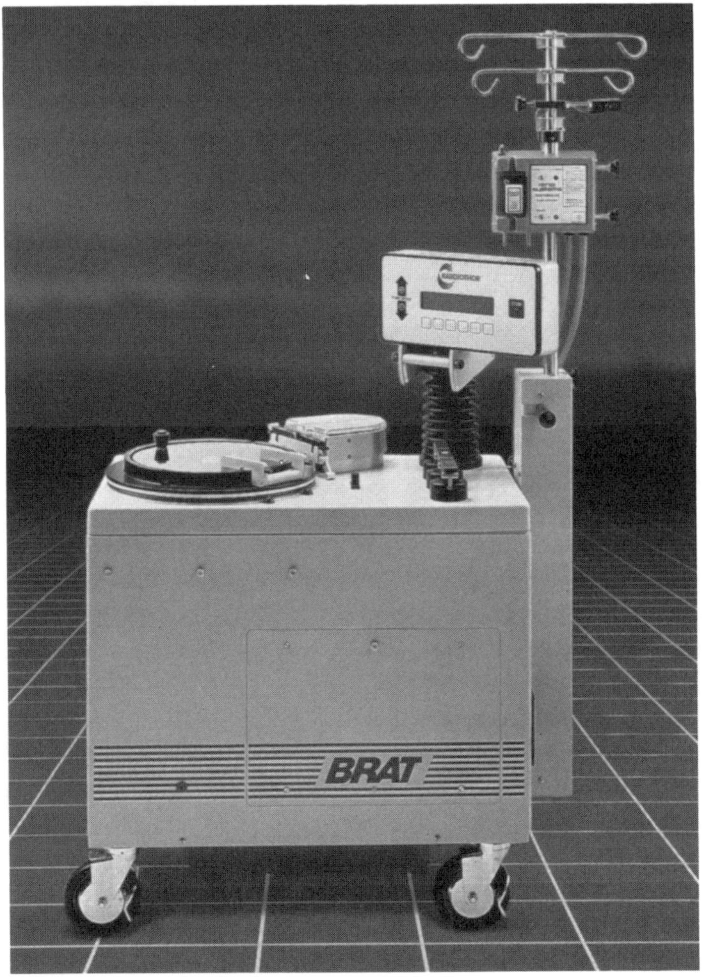

Figure 10.10 Autologous blood salvage machine. (Courtesy of Cobe Laboratories, Inc., Aravada, Colorado.)

Footnotes

[1]Harold A. Oberman, M.D., *Clinical Practice of Blood Transfusion*, eds. Lawrence D. Petz, M.D., and Scott N. Swisher, M.D. (New York: Churchill Livingstone, Inc., 1981), p. 9.

[2]Oberman, p. 11.

[3]*Ibid.*

[4]Jake Page, et al, *Blood: The River of Life*, (Washington, D.C.: U.S. News Books, 1981), p. 43.

[5]Oberman, p.13.

[6]Page, p.47.

[7]Oberman, p.15.

[8]R. Arnold Griswald, M.D., and Alvin B. Ortner, M.D., "The Uses of Autotransfusion in Surgery of the Serous Cavities," *Surgery, Gynecology, and Obstetrics*, 77 (January 1943).

ASSISTED CIRCULATION

CHAPTER ELEVEN

We have already mentioned that the heart's only function is to pump blood, that is, to move a fluid (romantic poets' notions to the contrary). It produces a flow (**cardiac output**) by ejecting part of its contents (**stroke volume** = amount of blood ejected per beat) during ventricular systole. **Ventricular systole** (the ejection phase) is followed by **ventricular diastole** (the filling phase). Together, they constitute one **cardiac cycle.** The **heart rate** (beats per minute) multiplied by the stroke volume equals **cardiac output** (the volume of blood pumped in one minute).

When left ventricular failure occurs, such as during or after an acute myocardial infarction, there is a decrease in stroke volume which causes a decrease in cardiac output. In other words, the cardiac output becomes inadequate to meet the body's needs. The determinants of stroke volume are **myocardial contractility** (the force of the muscular contraction or "squeeze" during systole), **preload** (the filling pressure or "stretch" during diastole), and **afterload** (the resistance or "impedance" against which the heart must empty its contents) (Figure 11.1). The greater the preload, the greater the stroke volume. This occurs to a point where the muscle is overstretched. At that point, further increases in filling pressure result in a decrease in cardiac output. This relationship is referred to as the "Frank-Starling Ventricular Function Curve," sometimes referred to as "Starling's Law of the Heart" (Figure 11.2).

The higher the resistance (afterload), the more work the heart performs to eject a given stroke volume. Circulatory assist devices are intended to improve the preload of the heart or to reduce the afterload.

With this background in mind, let's define a "circulatory assist device." Such a device is any mechanical apparatus designed to assist (not replace) the failing human heart

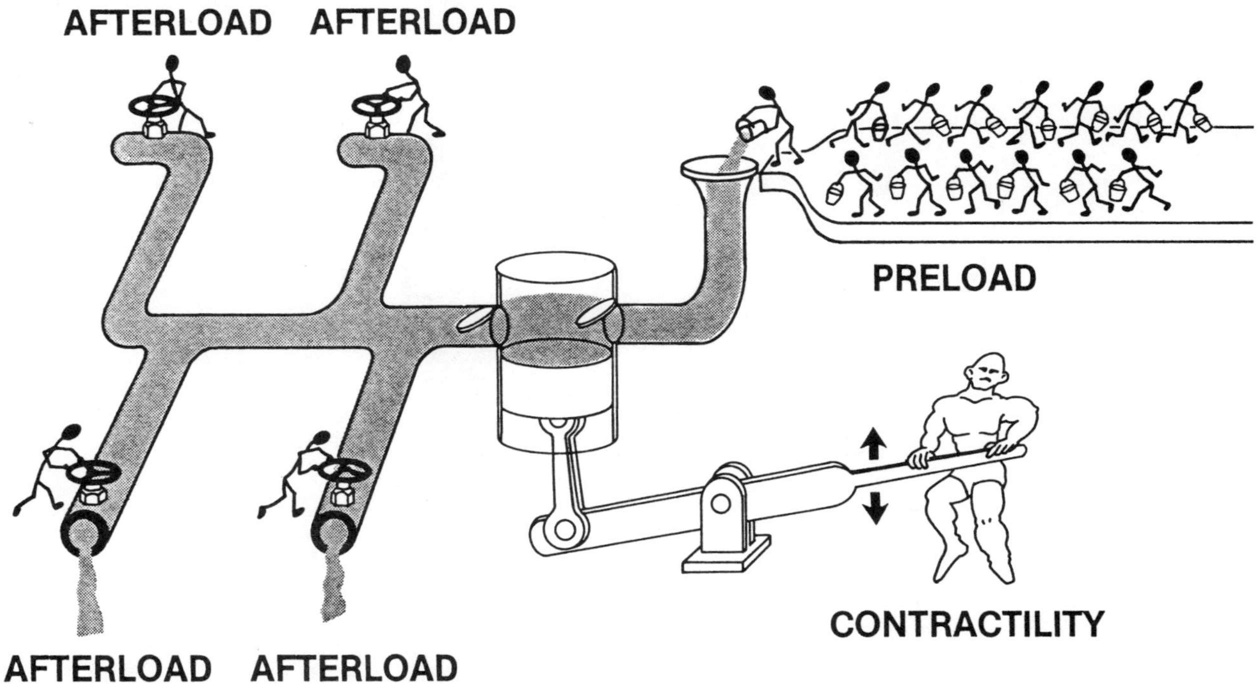

Figure 11.1 The determinants of cardiac function may be divided into preload, afterload, and contractility.

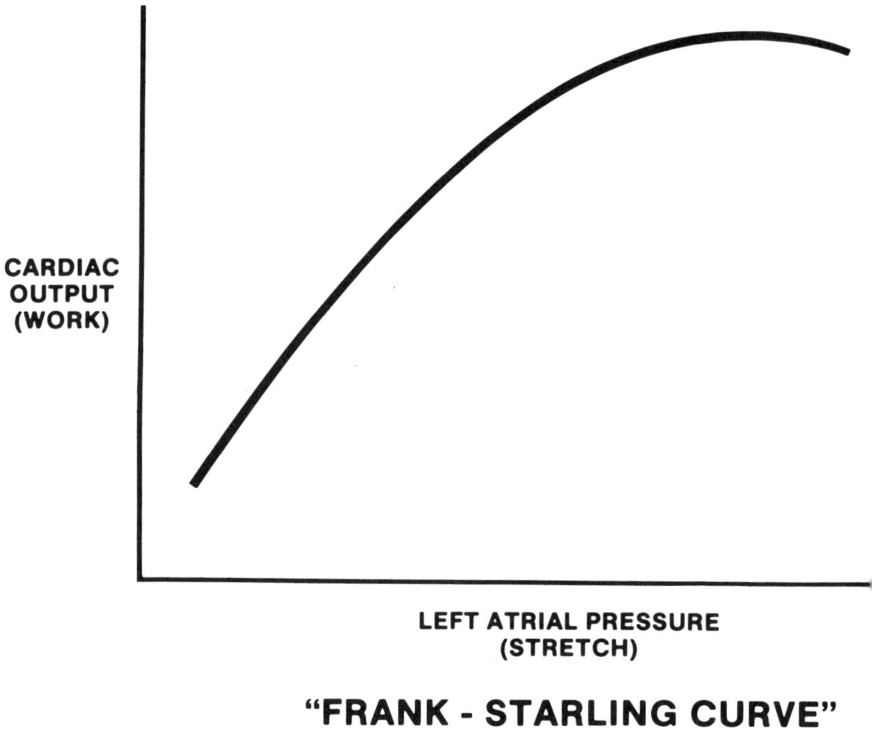
CARDIAC
OUTPUT
(WORK)
LEFT ATRIAL PRESSURE
(STRETCH)
"FRANK - STARLING CURVE"

Figure 11.2

until functional recovery can take place. Circulatory assist devices are essentially pumps that can take over the function or partial function of either or both ventricles. Some circulatory assist devices are blood pumps that reduce preload and afterload by physically supplying the energy (power) to pump blood; others, such as the intraaortic balloon pump, augment diastolic blood pressure by inflating during diastole and deflating just before the next systole (Figure 11.3). This action reduces afterload during cardiac failure by reducing the amount of resistance that the heart must pump against. Both kinds of circulatory assists, therefore, decrease the work that must be performed by the heart, reduce its oxygen consumption, and increase blood flow to the vital organs. Circulatory assist devices are used in cases where the patient cannot be weaned from cardiopulmonary bypass, despite pharmacological intervention or electrical pacemaking.

Partial Cardiopulmonary Bypass

Perhaps it will be helpful to define "*partial* cardiopulmonary bypass" by first defining "*total* cardiopulmonary bypass." During *total* cardiopulmonary bypass, all of the blood is diverted from the right side of the heart into the heart-lung machine, which assumes total cardiopulmonary function. This process empties the chambers of the heart in preparation for intracardiac surgery. During *partial* car-diopulmonary bypass, a portion of the blood is diverted to the heart-lung machine, while the remaining flow follows its normal circulatory path; for example, some blood still goes to the lungs and to the coronary circulation (Figure 11.4).

Usually, partial cardiopulmonary bypass is a temporary measure used following open heart surgery as a means to wean the patient from bypass. During this short period, the surgical team can normalize the patient's biochemical balance (acid base balance and electrolyte balance). Slowly, the heart is challenged to restart by gradually giving it more work to do. It is given more work by increasing the heart's filling pressure (preload). This is accomplished by

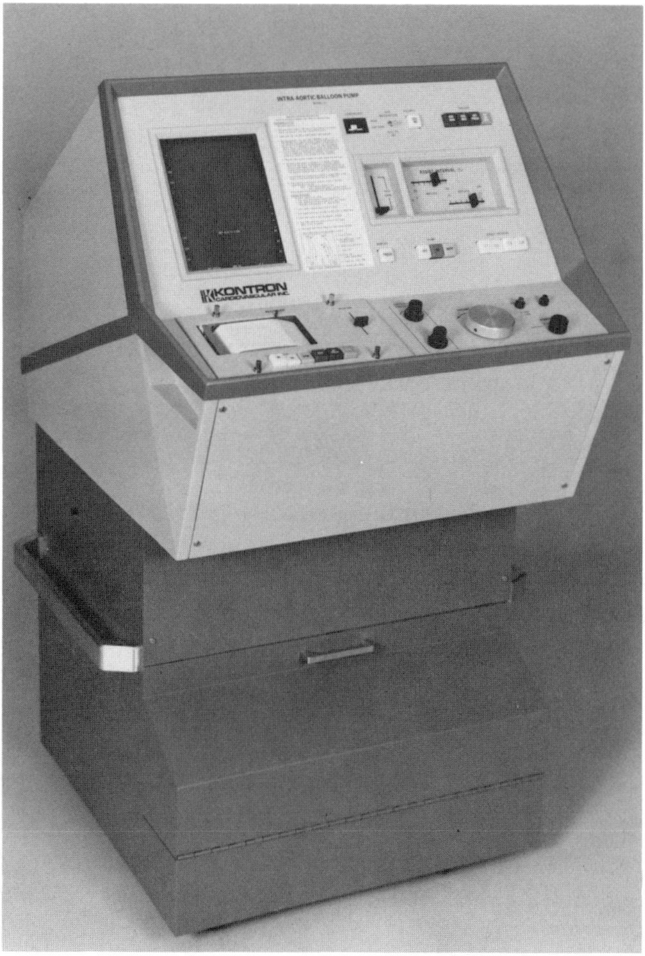

Figure 11.3 An intraaortic balloon pump control console. (Courtesy of Kontron Instruments, Everett, Massachusetts.)

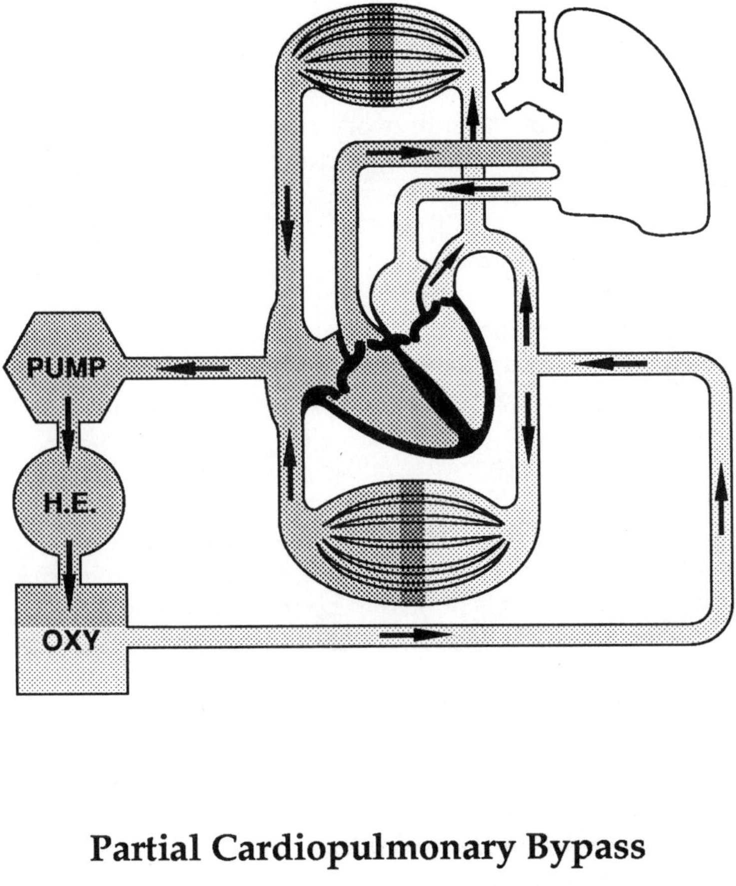

Partial Cardiopulmonary Bypass

Figure 11.4 During partial cardiopulmonary bypass, a portion of the blood is diverted to the heart-lung machine while the remaining flow follows its normal circulatory path.

transferring blood volume from the heart-lung machine to the patient while simultaneously reducing the blood flow through the heart-lung machine.

In about 5-10% of patients, the heart will not assume its function when challenged. Further support of circulation is needed and is provided by further partial cardiopulmonary bypass.

Partial cardiopulmonary bypass may be used for several hours following the open heart surgical procedure in an attempt to allow the heart to recover and to resume normal function. During partial cardiopulmonary bypass, the heart is still beating, but has little workload (filling pressure). Oxygenation may be improved, arrhythmias may be treated, blood and pharmacological agents (diuretics, cardiotonics, antiarrhythmics, additional anticoagulants) may be administered, and normal ventilation of the lungs may be started during this time.

There have been isolated instances reported in which patients were supported on partial cardiopulmonary bypass for several days. However, the heart-lung machine causes a significant physiological insult, so usually this kind of circulatory assist is limited to hours, rather than days. In those instances in which the cardiopulmonary bypass was extended for days, membrane oxygenators were employed because (as we mentioned in Chapter Five in the discussion of membrane oxygenators) this kind of artificial lung is much less traumatic to the formed elements of the blood (Figure 11.5).

Intraaortic Balloon Pump

One of the more common methods of treating "low output failure" (failure of the heart to pump an adequate blood flow) has been the use of the intraaortic balloon pump (Figure 11.7). This process is called "counterpulsation."

The intraaortic balloon is usually inserted in the thoracic aorta by way of the femoral artery. Once positioned, the balloon is inflated and deflated by an electromechanical balloon console (Figure 11.8). This mechanical action is

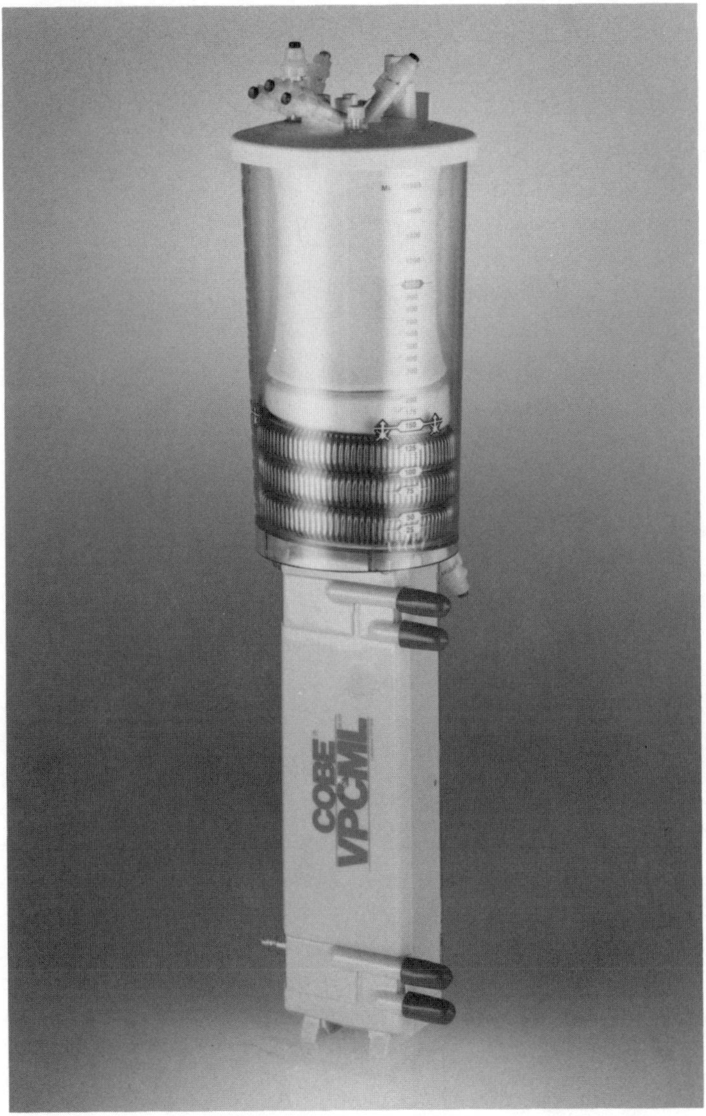

Figure 11.5 Membrane-type artificial lungs have been used for long-term circulatory support. (Courtesy of Cobe Laboratories, Aravada, Colorado.)

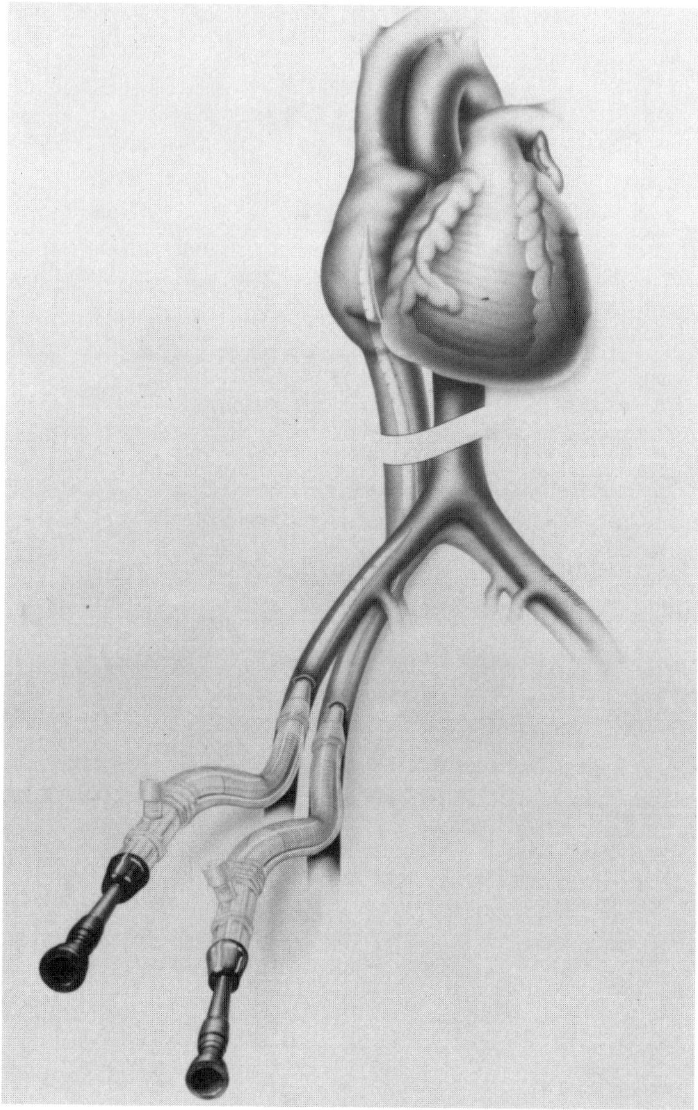

Figure 11.6 Cannulation of the inferior vena cava and aorta is made made passing cannulas into the femoral vessels. (Courtesy of Research Medical, Inc., Salt Lake City, Utah.)

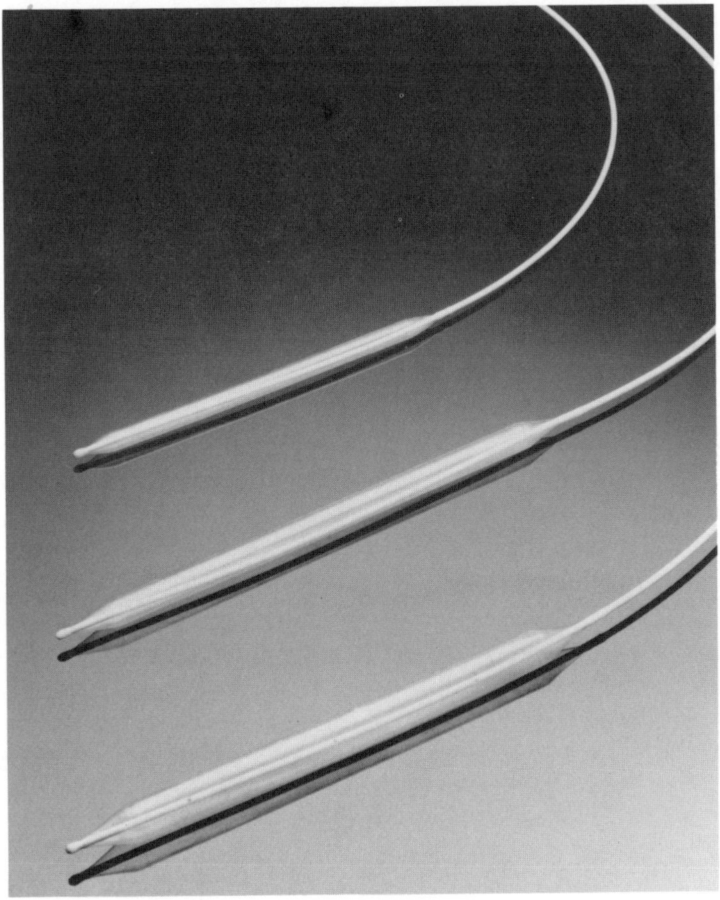

Figure 11.7 Intraaortic balloon pump catheters come in a variety of sizes. (Courtesy of Datascope, Paramus, New Jersey.)

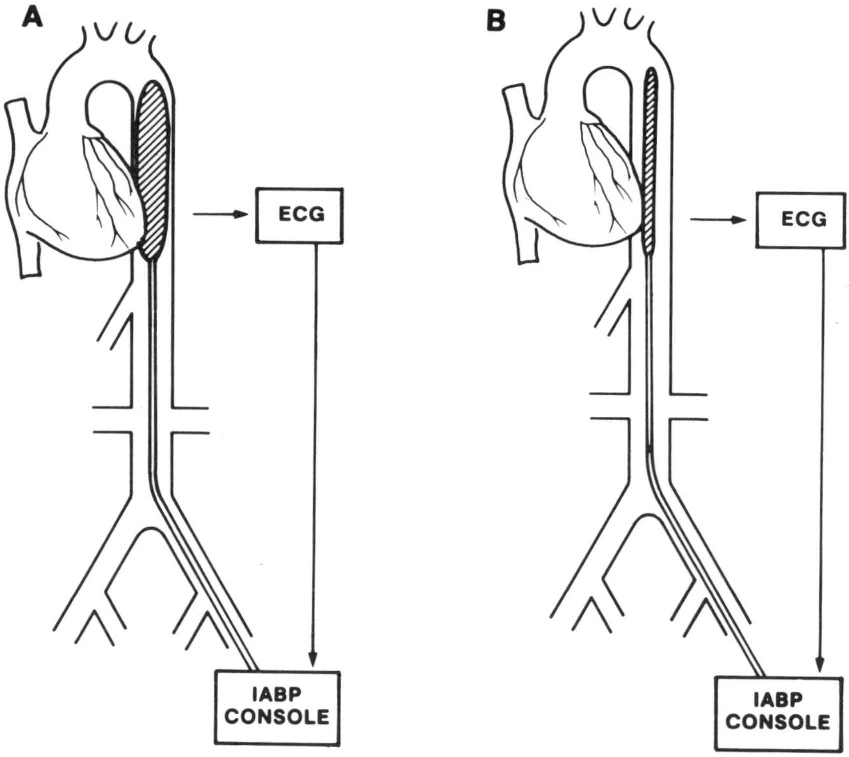

Figure 11.8 The intraortic balloon pump is synchronized by means of an electrocardiogram. **(A)** The balloon is inflated during ventricular systole. **(B)** The balloon is rapidly deflated prior to the next cardiac systole.

synchronized by means of an electrocardiogram.

Intraaortic balloons themselves are usually manufactured from medical grade polyurethane and are inflated with either helium or carbon dioxide, depending upon the manufacturer's recommendation. These gases are used because their density is less than compressed air. Since the flow of the gases creates less resistance, the gases can move in and out of the balloon more rapidly.

The intraaortic balloon is inflated during ventricular diastole. It is deflated just prior to ventricular systole. The balloon thus increases the arterial pressure during diastole (about 90% of coronary blood flow takes place during diastole). By deflating before the next systole, the balloon causes a reduction in afterload (in other words, there is a decrease in the hydraulic resistance that the heart must pump against).

Balloon pumps are used for a few days postoperatively in the patient with "low output failure" who cannot be weaned from cardiopulmonary bypass (Figure 11.9). The patient may be slowly weaned from the intraaortic balloon pump by either decreasing the volume in the balloon during inflation, or, more commonly, by inflating the balloon every other cardiac cycle, every fourth cardiac cycle, or every eighth cardiac cycle. It is commonly reported in the medical literature that balloon pumps may stabilize arrhythmias by increasing coronary blood flow and by reducing the amount of myocardial workload. Because balloon pumps increase the mean diastolic pressure, they also increase urinary output.

In addition to the treatment of "weaning problems," intraaortic balloon pumps have also been used in the treatment of cardiogenic shock secondary to acute myocardial infarction. Balloon pumps are also used to treat the "preinfarction angina syndrome" prior to myocardial revascularization surgery. When a patient is experiencing severe angina and has demonstrated coronary artery disease as evidenced by cardiac catheterization, the balloon pump may be used electively to reduce pain by increasing coronary blood flow

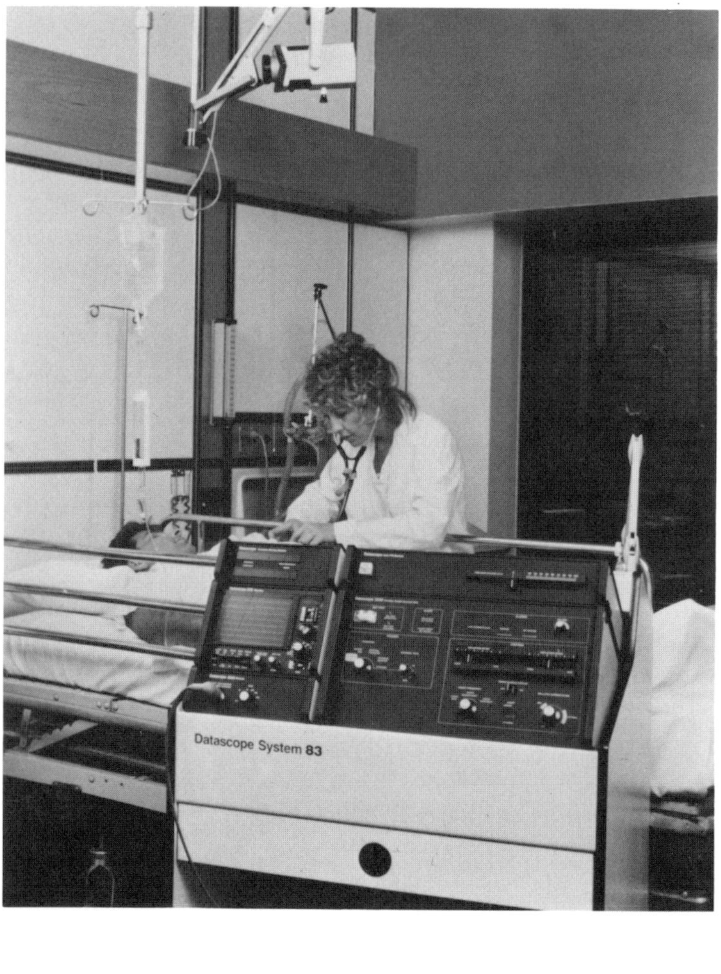

Figure 11.9 Intraaortic balloon pumps are used not only in surgery, but at the patient's bedside in the acute care unit setting. (Courtesy of Datascope, Paramus, New Jersey.)

and by reducing the heart's workload (afterload).

Intraaortic balloon pumps have a certain morbidity associated with their use. Many patients have experienced thromboembolic problems in their legs following the use of the intraaortic balloon pump. Some of these problems have resulted in leg amputations. Intraaortic balloon pumps are contraindicated in patients who have aortic valvular insufficiency. In these patients, when the balloon inflates during the augmented beat, increased pressure during diastole causes further regurgitation of the blood across the aortic valve, further compromising myocardial function. Also, in some patients, the physician may be unable to pass the balloon catheter through the leg artery because of the amount of atherosclerotic plaque in the artery. Another form of circulatory assist must be employed.

Left Heart Bypass

Extracorporeal circuits have been used for more than twenty years to bypass the left heart (Figure 11.10). Partial left heart bypass is successfully employed to wean patients from cardiopulmonary bypass following heart surgery when conventional support devices, such as intraaortic balloon pumps, partial cardiopulmonary bypass, and maximal drug therapy are unsuccessful.

A roller-type blood pump has been used to provide the external energy necessary to assume partial function of the left ventricle (Figure 11.11). However, direct cannulation of the left atrium when using a conventional roller pump poses some significant dangers. A conventional roller pump has the potential to generate high inlet negative pressures when the inlet is occluded. This could happen when the cannula is forced against the wall of the left atrium or when the atrium collapses around the cannula as a result of decreased circulating blood volume (hypovolemia). When the inlet is occluded in a high negative pressure situation, tearing of the atrial wall may result. In conjunction with the use of the roller pump, aspiration of air through the purse string at the cannulation site has also been reported, which

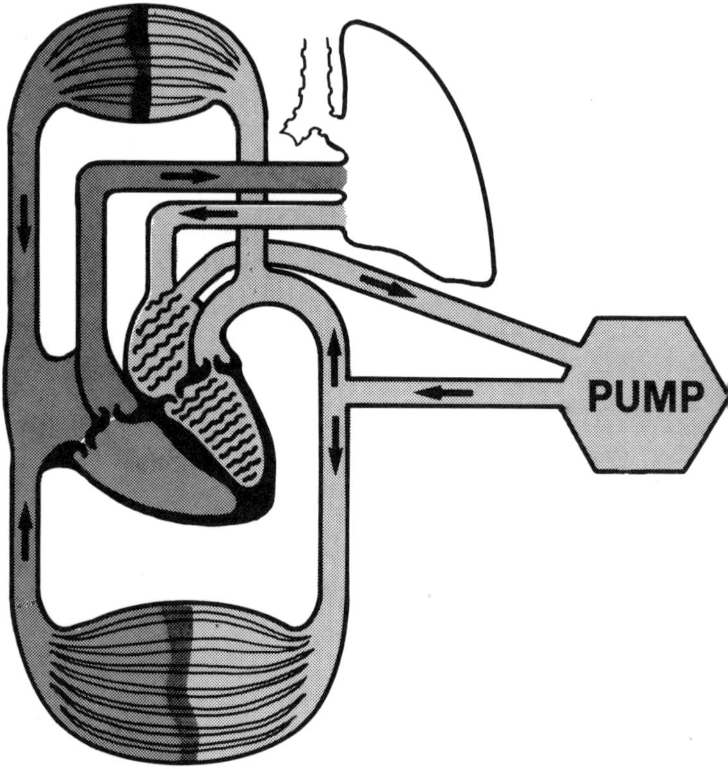

LEFT HEART BYPASS

Figure 11.10 During left heart bypass, a portion of the blood is diverted from the left heart and infused into the patient's arterial circulation.

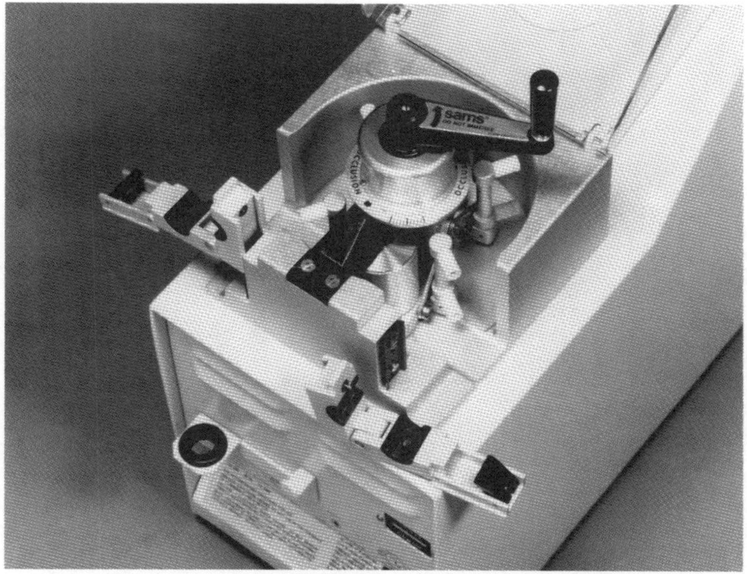

Figure 11.11 The roller-type blood pump has been used extensively for left heart bypass procedures. (Courtesy of Sarns, 3M Healthcare, Ann Arbor, Michigan.)

may cause an air embolism (Figure 11.12). To decrease these dangers (air embolism and physical tearing), a vented reservoir is often interposed between the left atrial cannulation site and the inlet of the roller blood pump. Of course, the perfusionist must pay careful attention to the level of blood in the reservoir so that air is not sucked into the circuit. (An unvented, bag-type reservoir may also be used.)

Left heart bypass (left atrium to aorta) has the physiological benefit of reducing left ventricular pre-load (filling pressure) while simultaneously assuming the "responsibility" for systemic blood flow. Hopefully, this will allow functional recovery of the heart.

An inflow cannula, designed by Dennis (an early investigator) and others, allows left heart bypass to be performed with a closed chest. In this procedure (described in 1961), the cannula is placed in the external jugular vein and advanced into the right heart. The curvature of the cannula guides it to the atrial septum. The cannula penetrates the septum, and is advanced into the left atrium where it can drain oxygenated blood into the inlet of the left heart bypass circuit.

Another cannulation technique (open chest) described by Litwak and others allows the arterial (aortic) cannula and the left atrial cannula to be sewn in place prior to left heart bypass. Following successful circulatory support, the cannulae are left in place as an implantable fixture. Obturators (devices to close the lumen) are inserted into both cannulae. The obturators can be removed to reinstitute left heart bypass. However, they are usually left in place to prevent blood clotting in the lumen of the cannula. The advantage of this system, of course, is not having to open the chest again to remove the cannulae.

There are other types of pumps other than the roller-type that are used in left heart bypass. They are the same types mentioned earlier that are used in standard bypass, i.e., reciprocating-type and centrifugal-type pumps. Some of these pumps (sac-type reciprocating pumps) will be discussed in the next chapter (Figures 11.13-11.17).

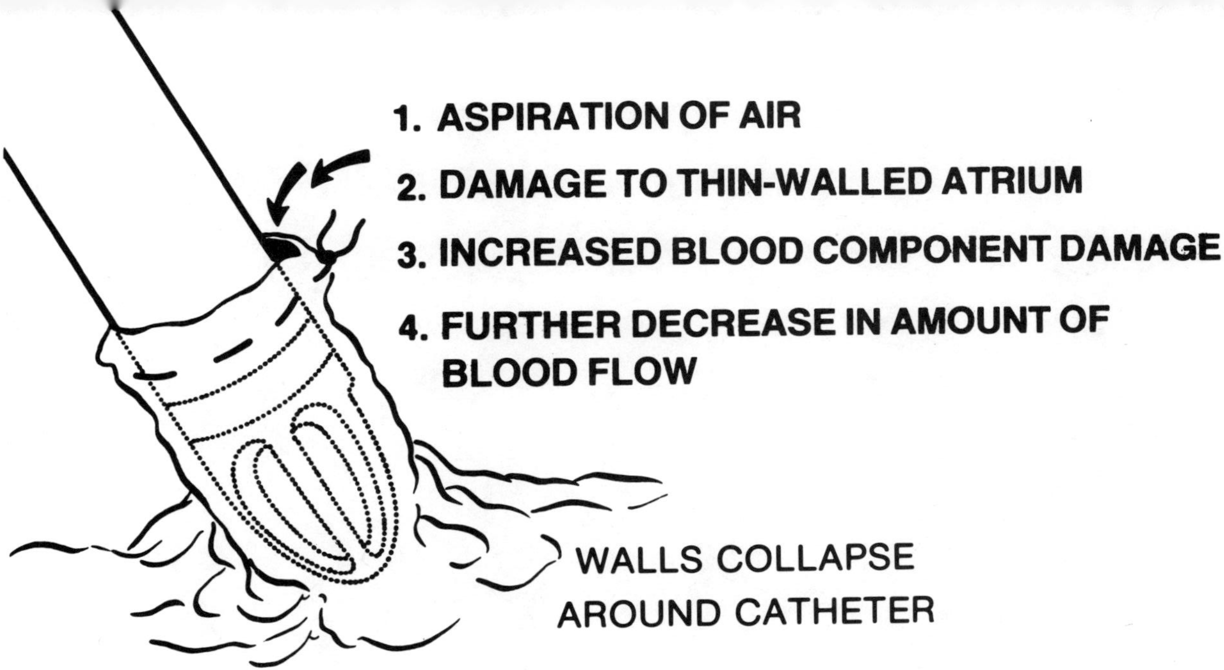

Figure 11.12 A number of problems have been associated with the use of a roller-type blood pump when direct atrial cannulation is employed.

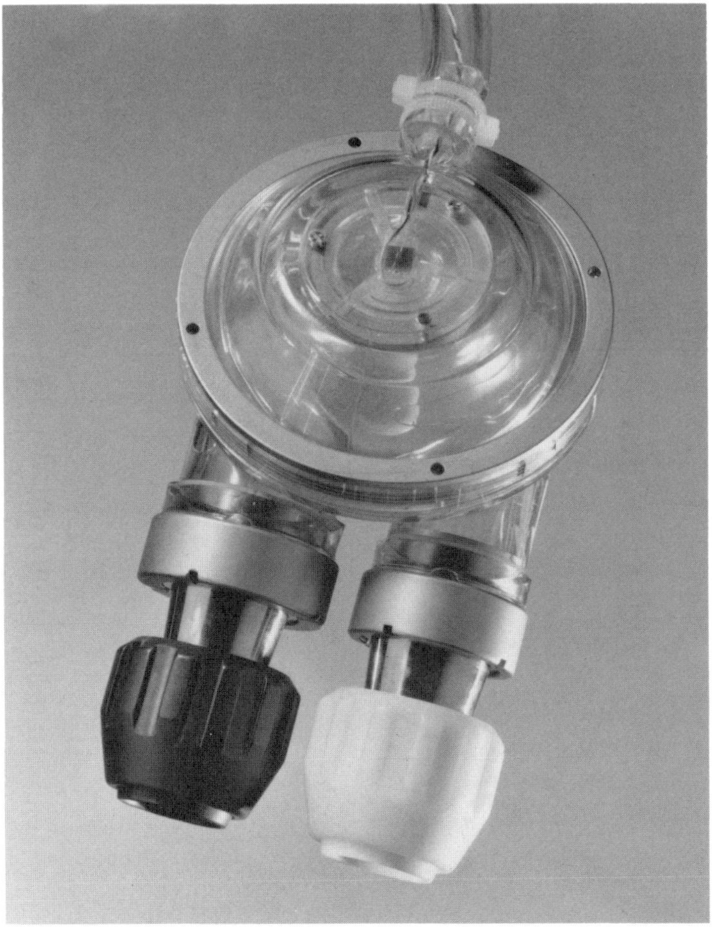

Figure 11.13 This external ventricular assist device was designed by Dr. William Pierce. (Courtesy of Sarns, 3M Healthcare, Ann Arbor, Michigan.)

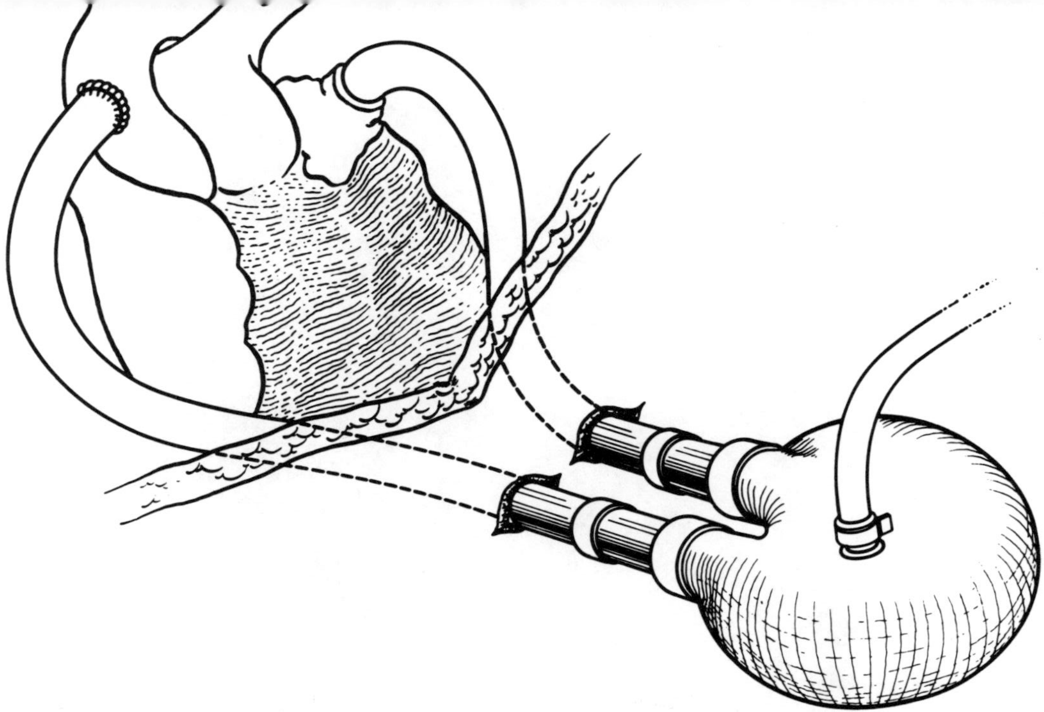

Figure 11.14 An external left ventricular assist device showing attachment to the heart.

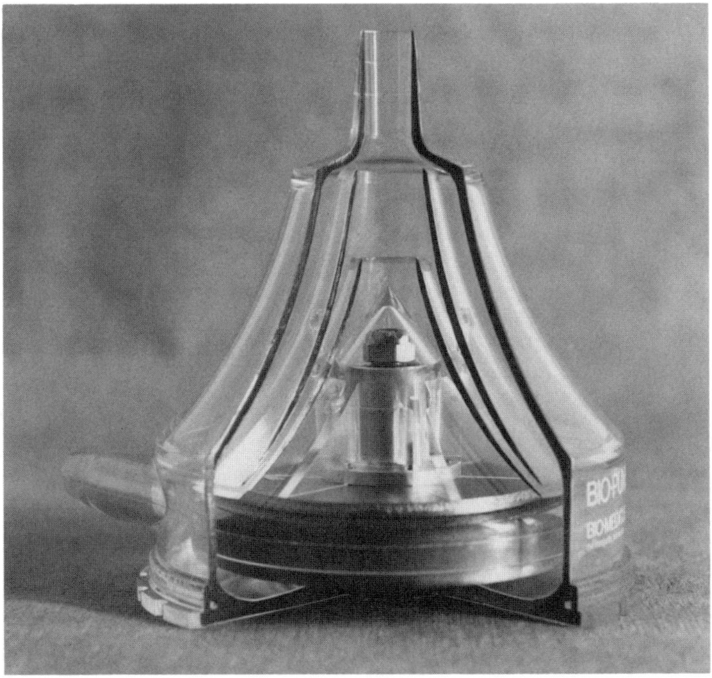

Figure 11.15 Centrifugal-type blood pumps have also been used for partial left heart bypass. Cutaway view. (Courtesy of Biomedicus, Minnetonka, Minnesota.)

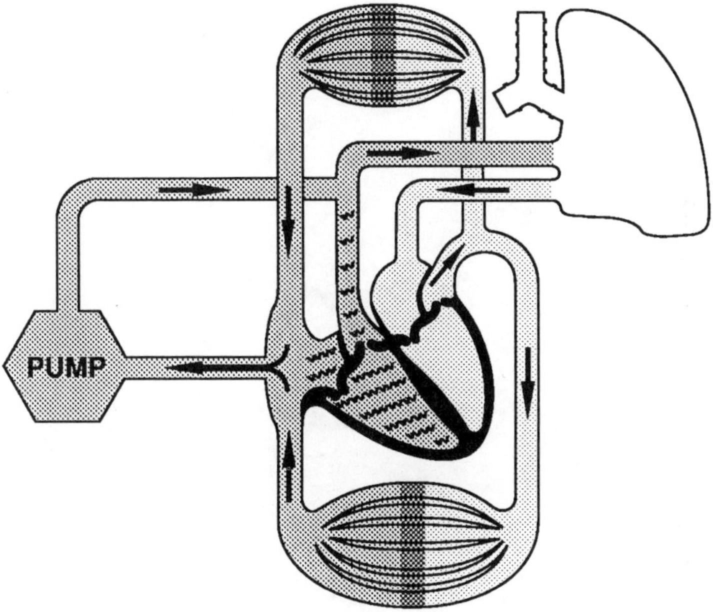

Right Heart Bypass

Figure 11.16 Bypass of the right heart has also been accomplished using various types of blood pumps.

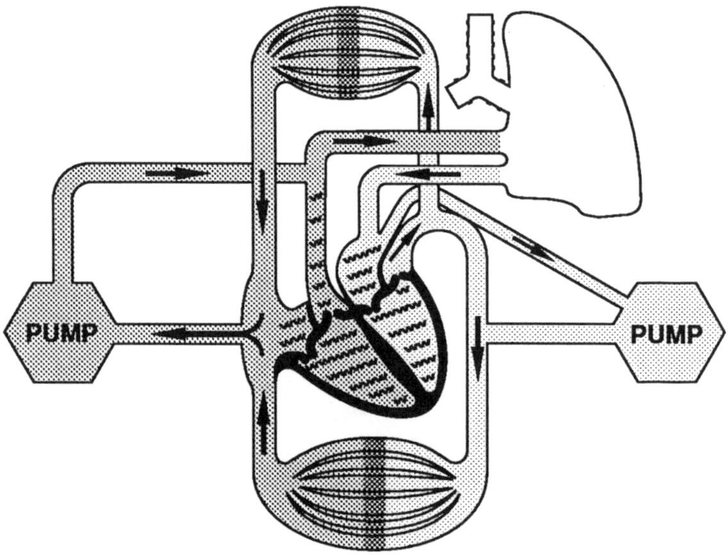

Right and Left Heart Bypass

Figure 11.17 Left and right heart bypass may be used simultaneously to support the failing circulation.

THE TOTAL ARTIFICIAL HEART

Chapter Twelve

In 1957, at the Cleveland Clinic, Dr. Tetsuzo Akutsu and Dr. Willem Kolff (Figure 12.1) implanted the first total artificial heart in a dog. The animal survived for 90 minutes.[1]

To design a pump to replace the human heart is a formidable task. There are many criteria which must be considered in the design of a totally implantable artificial heart. Ideally, the device should fit the anatomical space occupied by the natural heart and not impinge on the atria, the lungs, or the major blood vessels. The artificial heart must have an adequate cardiac output to meet the varying requirements of the body during exercise and rest. In other words, the artificial pump must be capable of variable cardiac output. Obviously, the artificial heart must be extremely reliable, durable, and easily sterilized. It must handle the blood in such a manner that the formed elements and the plasma proteins of the blood are not damaged. The heart must be of reasonable weight to avoid unnecessary movement and impingement upon surrounding structures. The heart must not generate excessive heat as a by-product of its own operation because such heat could elevate total body temperature and damage some blood elements. The materials from which the heart is fabricated must, of course, be extremely biocompatible. The artificial heart's power system should permit the patient to have maximum mobility. Again, one must remember that these criteria represent the "ideal" artificial heart and are not yet totally achieved.

One of the major problems experienced with artificial hearts has been the generation of thromboemboli. Prosthetic heart valves have a significant rate of thromboembolic complications. The artificial hearts each have four valves, thus increasing the exposure to thrombic formation. Too, the large blood-contact surface area of the artificial heart is a potential site for the formation of thrombi. The improved

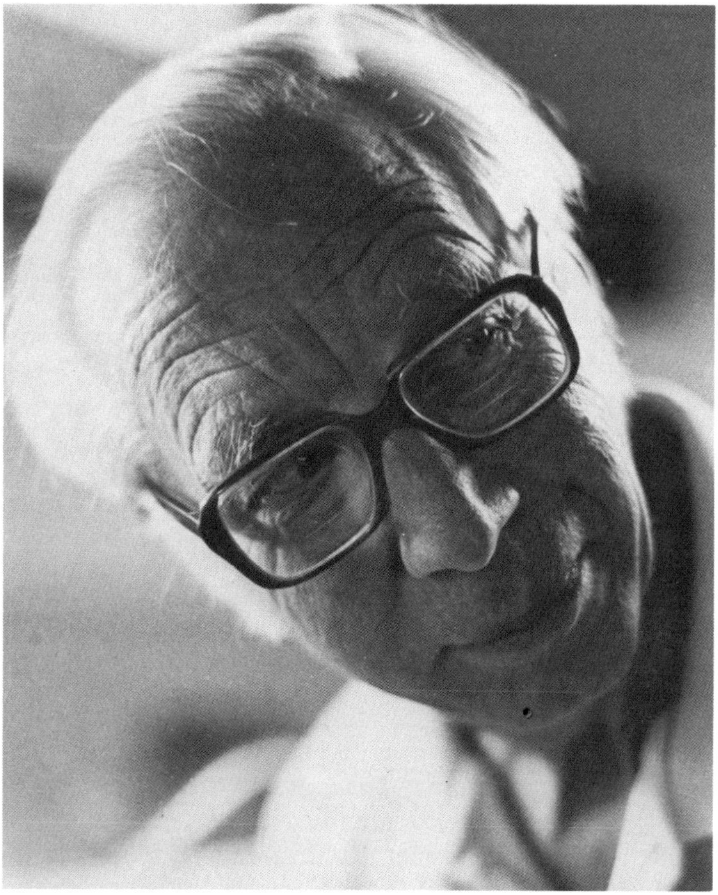

Figure 12.1 Dr. Willem Kolff, M.D., Ph.D., is known as "Father" of the artificial kidney and the artificial heart. (Photo courtesy of the Symbion Corporation, Salt Lake City, Utah.)

management of coagulation and the continuing development of better biocompatible surfaces will remedy many of these problems.

Materials

The first hearts which were designed by Drs. Akutsu and Kolff were fabricated from polyvinyl chloride. This plastic was easily available, relatively cheap, easy to work with, and had been widely used in other biomedical applications. Second generation artificial hearts were fabricated from silicone rubber compounds. The silicone models exhibited better blood handling characteristics than the polyvinyl chloride hearts but were less durable. The major components of most artificial hearts manufactured today are made from polyurethane. This plastic compound is extremely durable and biocompatible.

As mentioned early in this book, the natural human heart beats between 60 and 100 times per minute. In a year, it beats approximately 50 million times. Thus, the materials from which an artificial heart is fabricated must withstand the constant flexion imposed upon them by blood pumping requirements. The durability of the artificial heart is an unresolved problem. Most of the hearts in use today have a design goal of only a few years of operation (Figure 12.2).

Drive Systems

The total artificial heart first implanted by Akutsu and Kolff in 1957 was operated by air pressure. Such pneumatic pumps are very reliable, do not generate heat as a byproduct of their operation, and are light weight. Compressed air is readily available as a power source. The major disadvantage of such a system is the need for the two relatively large percutaneous air lines which are connected from the heart to an external drive system. The opening where the air lines penetrate the skin is obviously a potential site for infection and has posed continual problems for the proponents of pneumatically-driven hearts. However, new design changes, and devices such as Teflon skin buttons (which

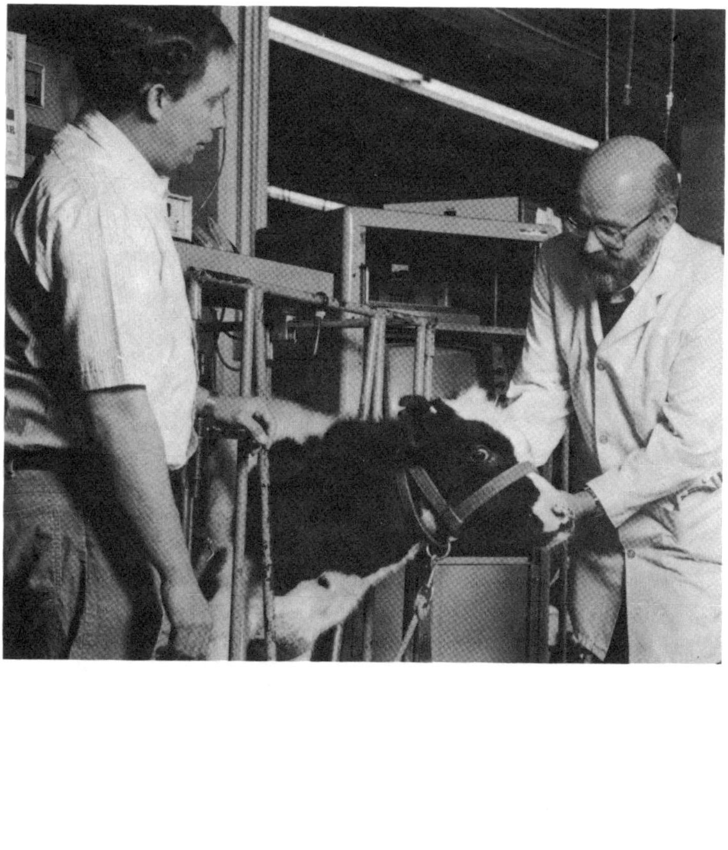

Figure 12.2 Don Olson, D.V.M., and Engineer Steven Neilson are pictured with a calf whose circulation is totally supported by a total artificial heart at the University of Utah. (Photo courtesy of the Symbion Corporation, Salt Lake City, Utah.)

encourage tissue ingrowth) through which the air lines pass, are reducing the number of problems caused by infections. We expect that this kind of problem will cease to be a major one in the near future. The other disadvantage of the pneumatic drive system is the limited mobility afforded the patient. However, drive systems are becoming increasingly portable as evidenced by the units used by the patients of Dr. William DeVries in Kentucky. Such portable systems have permitted patients to leave the hospital or the home environment—away from the large power consoles—for several hours.

Several systems have been designed that employ electrical power. However, such systems have not been implanted in a human because they have not proven as reliable as the pneumatic systems.

The Westinghouse Corporation, with the cooperation of the federal government and scientists at the University of Utah under the direction of Dr. Kolff, designed a nuclear-powered artificial heart in 1975. However, the size and weight of the heart, in addition to the potential political and security problems of radioactivity, caused work to stop on this project for the time being.

All of the heart designs at the time of this writing that have been implanted in human beings have been pneumatically driven.

Human Implant Experience: A "Bridge to Transplantation"

In 1969, Dr. Denton Cooley implanted a total artificial heart designed by Domingo Liotta in a patient who had undergone a resection of a left ventricular aneurysm and who had irreversible cardiac decompensation. The patient could not be weaned from cardiopulmonary bypass, so the total artificial heart procedure was attempted. This implant was the first total artificial heart implant made in a human being. The device served as a "bridge" for cardiac transplantation and kept the patient alive for 64 hours until a donor heart was found. The transplant functioned for an additional 32 hours until the patient died of pneumonia.

In July, 1981, Dr. Cooley implanted another pneumatically-driven artificial heart designed by Dr. Akutsu. This artificial heart was used for 27 hours as a temporary measure until a donor heart was available.

Dr. Cecil Vaughn (Figure 12.3) and Dr. Jack Copeland implanted a pneumatically-driven artificial heart designed by Dr. Kevin Cheng as a bridge to transplantation in March, 1985 at the University of Arizona in Tucson. The patient was a 32 year old man whose transplanted heart had failed because of hyperacute rejection. The so-called "Phoenix Heart" functioned well for 11 hours until a new donor heart could be transplanted. This patient died a few days following the last transplant. The young man became the first patient in history to have four hearts—one natural, one artificial, and two transplants.

It should be noted that all of the patients described here were desperately ill. And although the length of time that they survived was not long, these experiences have demonstrated the feasibility of using the total artificial heart as a bridge to transplantation. The state-of-the-art in heart replacement is still the donor heart transplant. However, donor heart transplantation can rarely be used as an emergency procedure. The total artificial heart does provide an "off-the-shelf" solution for circulatory support until a donor heart transplant can be performed.

Human Implant Experience: Permanent Implants

Dr. William DeVries implanted a total artificial heart (Jarvik-7) in the chest of a 61 year old dentist, Dr. Barney Clark, in December of 1982 (Figure 12.4). The procedure was performed as a permanent replacement for Dr. Clark's damaged natural heart. He was terminally ill. The artificial heart pumped blood for his body for 112 days.

Subsequently, Dr. DeVries has implanted the Jarvik-7 in several patients at the Humana Heart Institute in Louisville, Kentucky. None of the patients who received total artificial hearts were candidates for donor heart transplantation. As a result of these limited "experiments," the

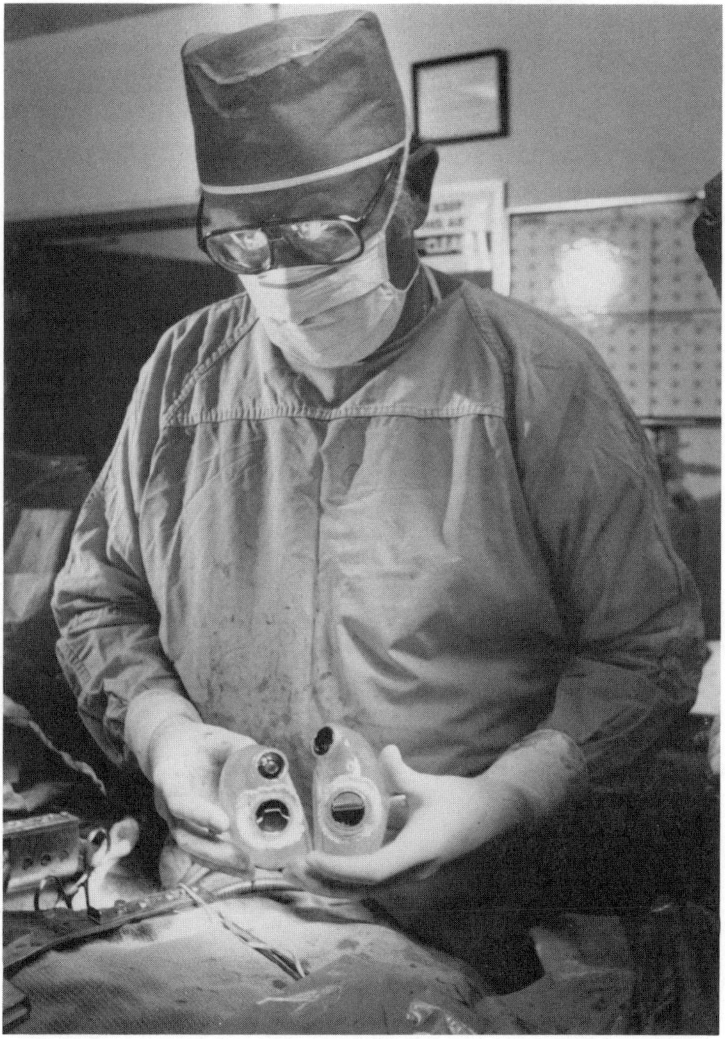

Figure 12.3 Cecil C. Vaughn, M.D., is pictured with the "Phoenix Heart," designed by Kevin Cheng, D.D.S. (Photo courtesy of St. Luke's Medical Center, Phoenix, Arizona.)

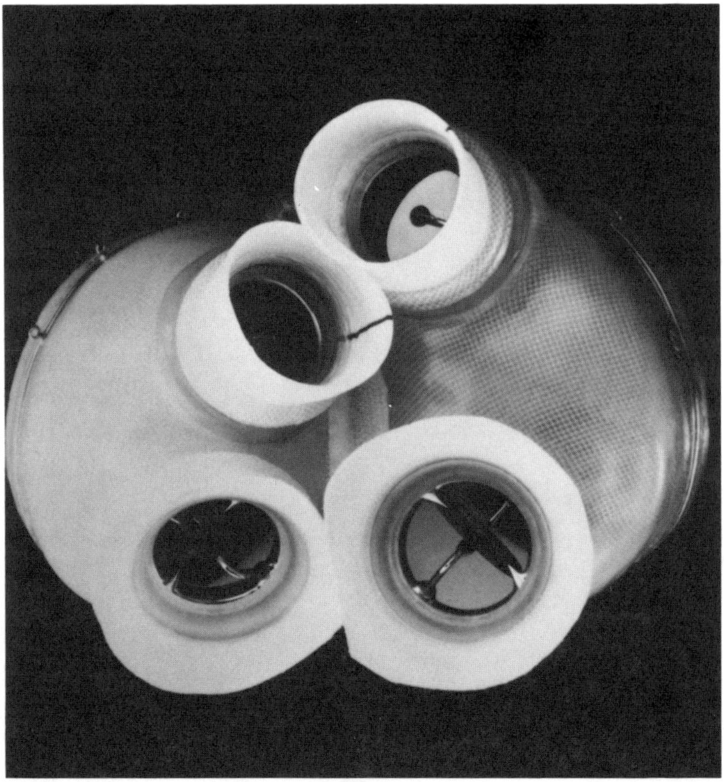

Figure 12.4 The "Jarvik-7" was used by William DeVries, M.D., as a permanent replacement for a damaged natural heart. (Courtesy of the Symbion Corporation, Salt Lake City, Utah.)

plantation. As a result of these limited "experiments," the use of total artificial hearts in the future is very encouraging. However, ethical and economic questions remain to be answered before the use of the total artificial heart is widespread.

Summary

Most artificial hearts that have been implanted so far have been driven by compressed air. These kinds of artificial hearts are designed with both a right-sided pump (which pumps blood to the lungs) and a left-sided pump which pumps oxygenated blood received from the lungs out to the systemic circulation. These pumps are classified as the reciprocating type, as described earlier in this text. These pumps operate in this fashion: each side of the heart alternately fills and empties by the back-and-forth displacement of an air sac. Valves are required at both the inlets and the outlets of the ventricles. Thus far, all of the valves that have been used clinically have been FDA-approved prosthetic heart valves such as those used in prosthetic heart valve replacement operations. Some mobility has been gained by artificial heart patients by means of portable battery-powered compressed air drives. However, the present designs still require that a patient be tethered to the drive system by air lines that are about 8 feet long. At this writing, a compressed air supply as well as portable gas cylinders (used as a backup in the event of electrical or mechanical failure) must be located adjacent to the patient's living quarters.

Some scientists predict that in the forseeable future a workable artificial heart will be designed with its own internal energy supply. Until that time, however, a patient tethered to an air-driven artificial heart is not necessarily bedridden or hospitalized. According to Dr. Kolff, a patient can be out of bed in a few days after the implantation and can be "... more mobile than a patient who is confined to a wheelchair" (Figures 12.5-12.8).

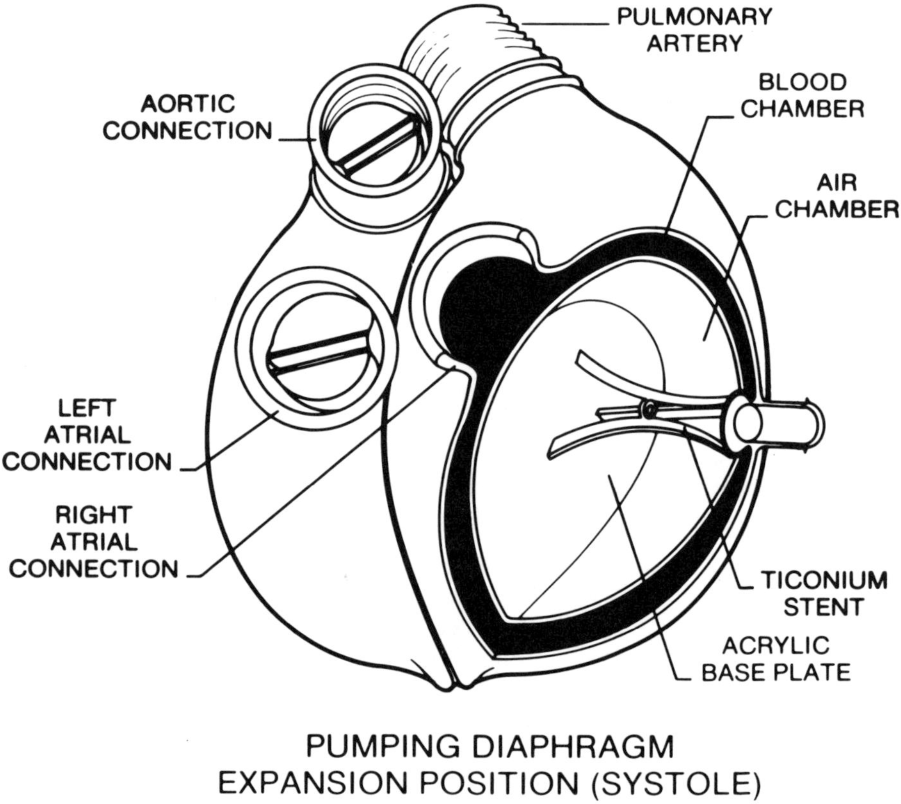

Figure 12.5 A cutaway section of the "Phoenix Heart."

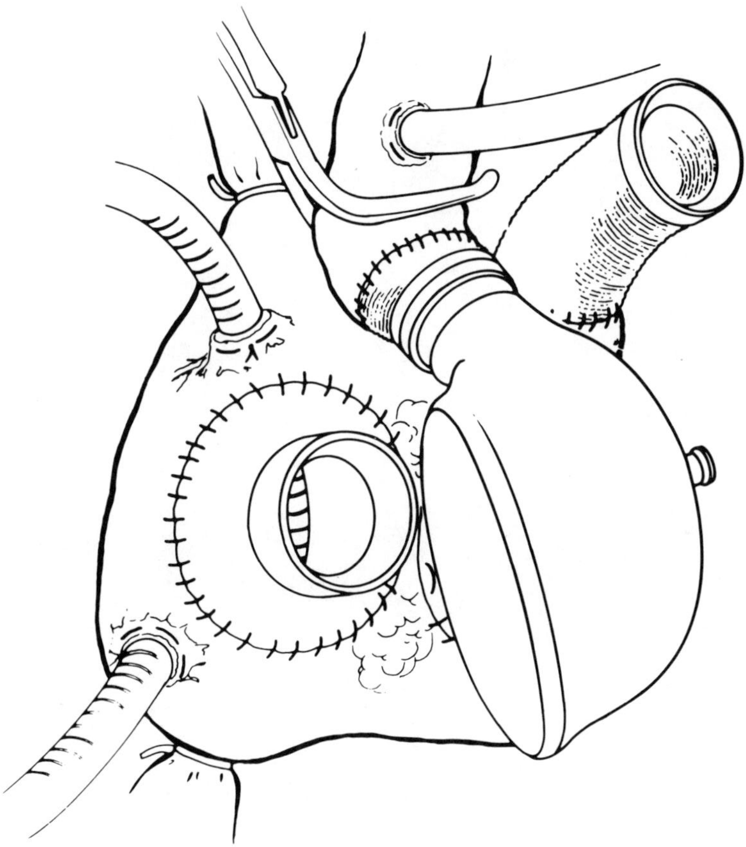

Figure 12.6 The left side of the "Phoenix Heart" is shown in place.

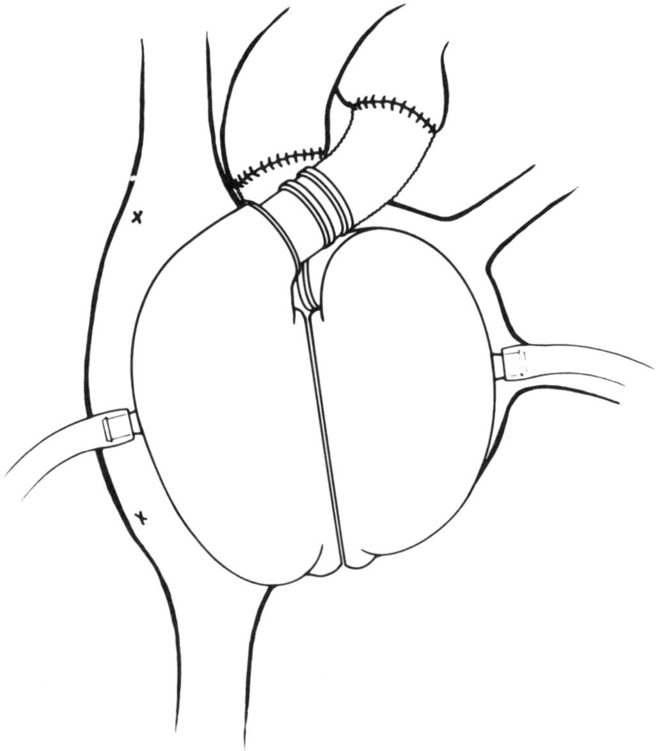

Figure 12.7 Both sides of the "Phoenix Heart" are attached in this illustration.

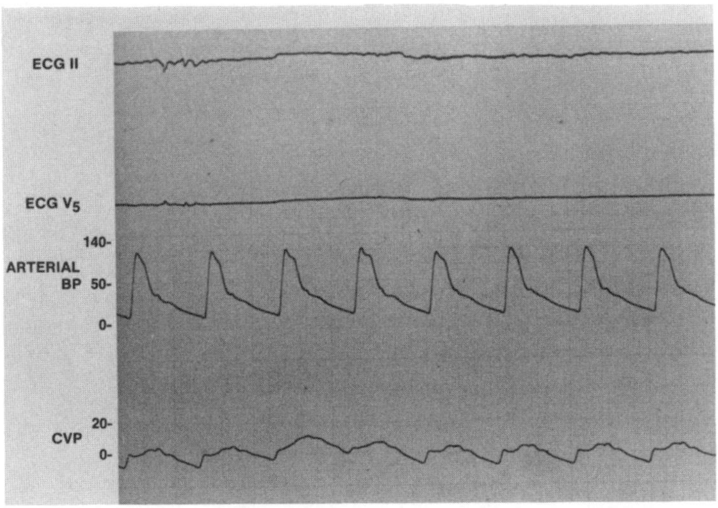

Figure 12.8 The arterial blood pressure and central venous pressure are depicted in actual use in the patient with the "Phoenix Heart." Note the "flat" ECG.

Footnotes

[1]Dr. Willem Kolff was raised and educated in the Netherlands. He is most famous, perhaps, for his work as the inventor of the artificial kidney. However, it is the authors' shared opinion that he should also be known as "Father" of the total artificial heart because he has been the "driving force" behind most of the many developments that have been made in this kind of research. Kolff left the Cleveland Clinic in 1967 to head the Artificial Organs Division, University of Utah.

POSTOPERATIVE EFFECTS OF OPEN HEART SURGERY

CHAPTER THIRTEEN

As previously discussed in the section concerning the pathophysiology of cardiopulmonary bypass, there are many deviations from normal physiology that occur during bypass. In this chapter, we intend to outline the major postoperative complications and morbidity that may follow open heart surgery. Obviously, not all of these complications are caused directly by cardiopulmonary bypass. E. Converse Pierce II, M.D., expresses it this way: "The ultimate objective of extracorporeal circulation is to provide normal organ perfusion while the surgeon has optimal conditions..." to perform cardiac operations. "Present day open heart surgery is, consequently, not ideal and is successful only if the organ derangements produced during the procedures are merely reversible."[1]

Psychological & Neurological Complications

Patients who have just undergone open heart surgery immediately have major physical and psychological changes in their lives. Frequently, the otherwise healthy patient may have just discovered the presence of this life-threatening disease—often just a day or two before surgery. The result of the medical treatment and the disease state may result in a severe loss of independence. The patient is dependent upon the judgement and the medical skills of the open heart team. The patient is dependent upon an intimidating, complex array of equipment found in the surgical suite and in the intensive care unit. The patient becomes dependent upon others for financial aid—an insurance company, an institution, or a relative, perhaps. The patient may have to depend on others to continue work responsibilities—run a business or provide family income.

The anxiety and fear of one's potential death is extremely stressful. Worrying about the effect of one's death upon the family may produce addition psychological distress.

An intensive care unit itself may have a negative psychological impact (Figure 13.1). There are many interruptions in the operation of a patient's normal biological time clock. Patients often become confused and have difficulty distinguishing night from day. Machine noise, strange voices and sounds, telephones, and monitor alarms constantly interrupt sleep patterns. All these factors, together with the fact that the patient is usually on several medications, among them narcotics, may considerably alter normal sensory input. Collectively, the psychological disorders produced by all of these changes are known as "postoperative psychosis." Accompanying this kind of disorder may be periods of total amnesia and episodes involving delusions, hallucinations, and confusion. It should be noted that this kind of psychosis is not exclusive to open heart surgery but also occurs following other kinds of major surgery. Postoperative psychoses may also be caused by drugs, hepatic or renal insufficiency, cerebral vascular insufficiency, CNS trauma, and a number of other reasons.

Whether a postoperative psychosis is of organic or psychological origin may be difficult to determine and is the subject for another book. However, it may be safe to say that all open heart surgery patients experience some kind of psychological abnormality. In most cases, the abnormality is mild-to-severe depression. When considered carefully, even the state invoked during the post-anesthesia period is abnormal.

Many neurological abnormalities following open heart surgery are relatively minor and transient, such as visual defects (e.g., blind spots), memory lapses, slurred speech, and minor paralysis. Some neurological abnormalities may be severe and even life-threatening, such as total paralysis or a comatose state.

What causes these neurological abnormalities? Many are caused by embolic phenomena. For example, the transient blind spots experienced by many open heart patients

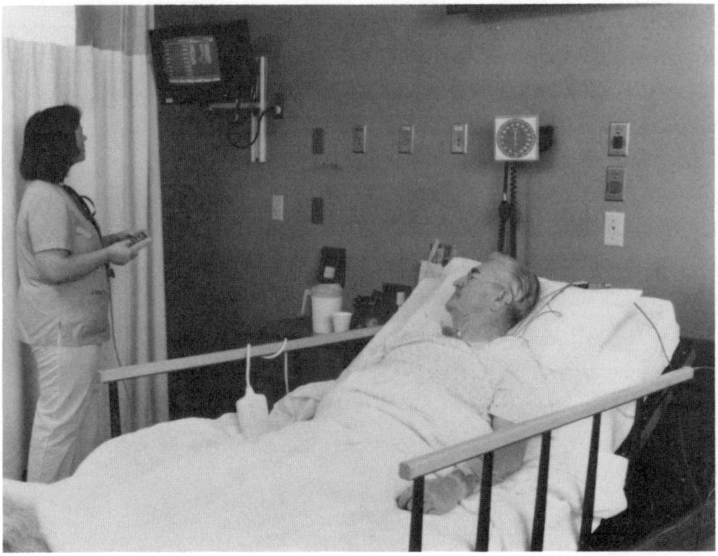

Figure 13.1 The intensive care unit can cause abnormalities in a patient's sensory responses.

are probably caused by micro-emboli in the retinal blood vessels. As mentioned in Chapter Seven, atherosclerotic plaque material may be dislodged during open heart surgery and be swept into the arterial circulation to the brain, causing a cerebral vascular accident that could result in paralysis or prolonged unconsciousness.

Thus far, we have mentioned embolic problems caused by thrombi or debris. In addition to these "solid" emboli, air emboli can cause minor-to-catastrophic problems. For example, air may remain in a heart chamber following a cardiotomy. This residual air may be released as emboli that migrate to the brain and block blood vessels of varying sizes. Bubble-type oxygenators at times may "shower" the patient with micro bubbles. These bubbles have been identified with ultrasonic detectors (counters). The effects of such an incidence are not well understood; however, one may assume that such a "shower" is not conducive to good health.

A major (but infrequent) catastrophe can occur during extracorporeal bypass if the oxygenator is allowed to run dry and air is pumped to the patient. The resulting massive air embolus may cause severe neurological damage or death.

Cardiac Failure (or "pump" failure)

We have discussed the treatment of cardiac failure (associated with open heart surgery) by means of mechanical circulatory assist in Chapter Eleven. Low output cardiac failure (including failure associated with arrhythmias) is the most common cause of postoperative mortality in the open heart surgical patient. The causes of cardiac failure are many, and many causes are not clearly understood.

One cause of postoperative cardiac failure is incomplete correction of an intracardiac defect, such as is found in the correction of congenital heart defects when the correction is performed in stages.

Another cause may be found during coronary bypass procedures when the surgeon is unable to graft the intended vessels because of their small size or because of the unrecognized severity of the disease process prior to surgery.

Yet another cause of cardiac failure is inadequate myocardial protection. Inadequate myocardial protection may be caused by an extended ischemic time or by conditions caused by the disease itself that increase ischemic time (e.g., finding an unexpected number of small vessels that must be grafted during aortocoronary bypass surgery).

Low output failure may also be caused by the type of pericardial tamponade that is caused by blood clots (resulting from seepage) that collect in the pericardial sac following open heart surgery. The clots surround the heart (specifically the atria) and prevent the heart from filling properly. This condition is characterized by high central venous pressure and low arterial blood pressure. In other words, the clots interfere with the adequate preloading of the heart during diastole which, in turn, causes low output failure. This kind of tamponade is a common reason why patients must often be returned to the operating room for reexploration after an open heart procedure.

At this point, it is necessary to mention arrhythmias in connection with cardiac failure. Strictly speaking, any prolonged arrhythmia is a "failure of the pump" and in time may cause cardiac failure. Some arrhythmias, such as a single premature ventricular beat; a single premature atrial contraction; or a mild, transient bradycardia or tachycardia, do not cause cardiac failure. Some arrhythmias, notably ventricular fibrillation, ventricular tachycardia, and ventricular standstill, may cause sudden and life-threatening cardiac failure (Figures 13.2-13.5).

Arrhythmias are caused by myocardial damage (such as the damage caused by a myocardial infarct or damage caused in an attempt to repair a congenital heart defect), by electrolyte imbalance, or by an interruption of coronary blood flow.

Electrolyte imbalance may be caused by increased diuresis during the operation. This state of imbalance is

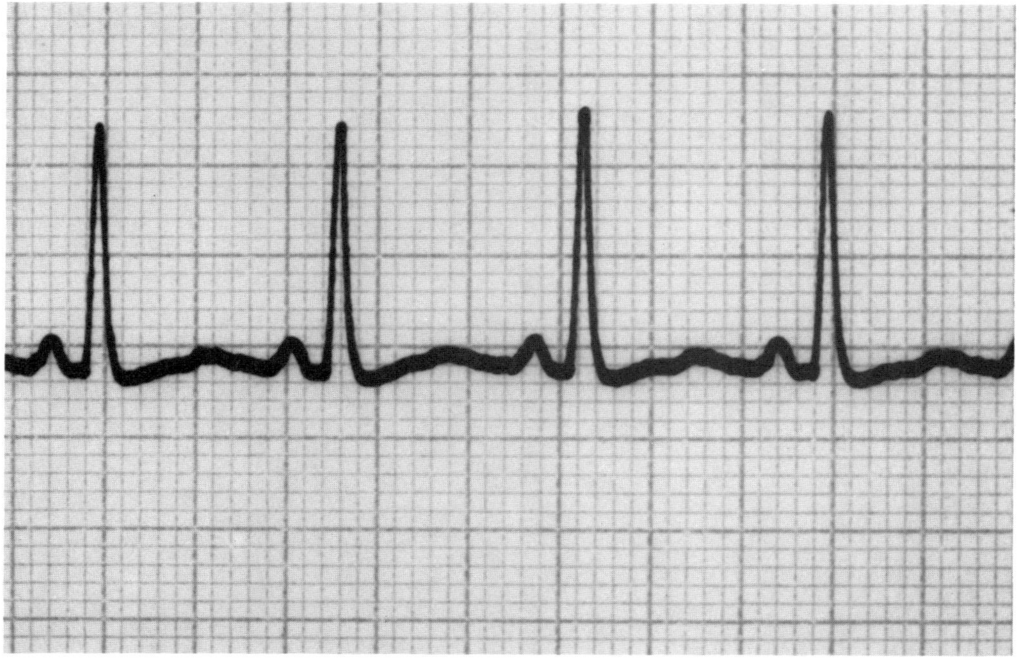

Figure 13.2 Rhythm strip of sinus rhythm.

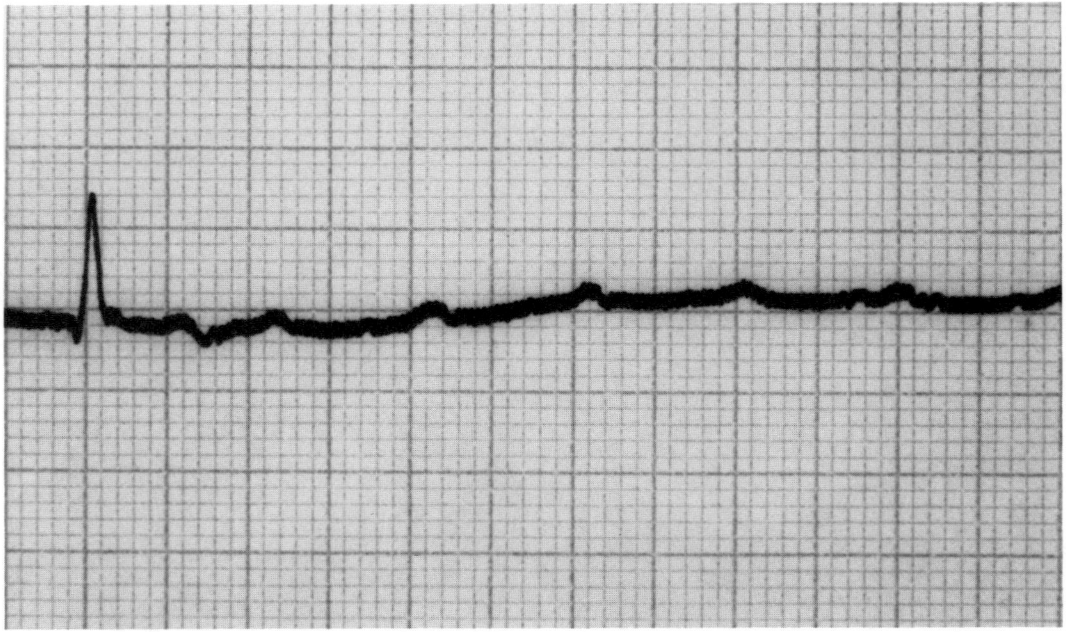

Figure 13.3 Rhythm strip showing one ventricular beat followed by total heart block.

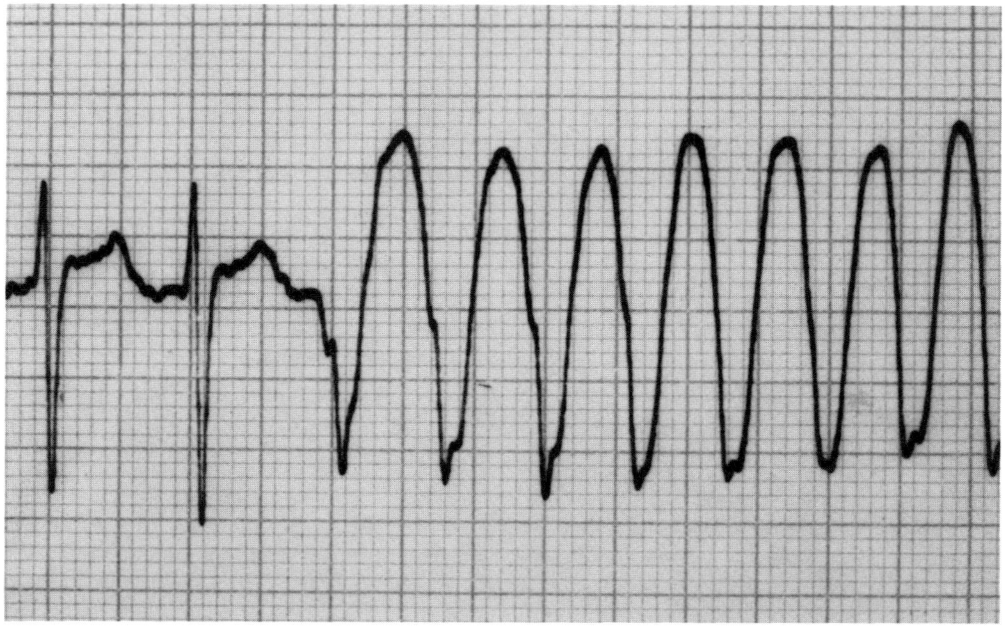

Figure 13.4 Two ventricular beats followed by ventricular tachycardia.

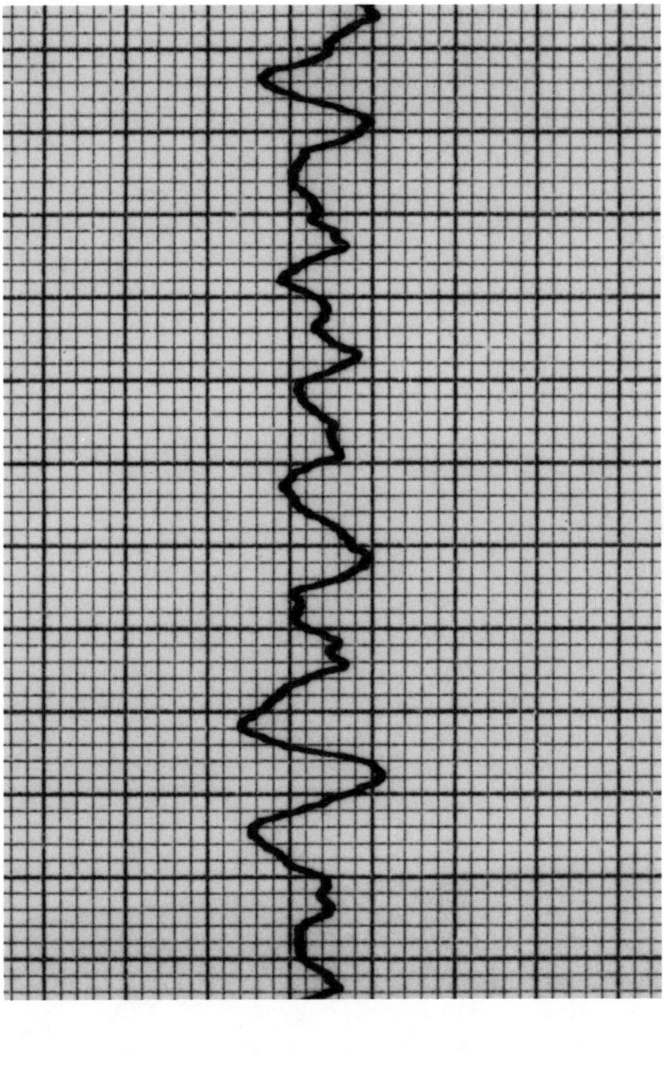

Figure 13.5 Ventricular fibrillation.

increased by the hemodilution that occurs as a matter of course with priming of the heart lung machine and with the addition of cardioplegic solutions to the circulation. This kind of imbalance "dilutes" the electrolyte ions. Decreased diuresis may also cause electrolyte imbalance by "concentrating" the electrolyte ions. The myocardium becomes particularly irritable and arrhythmia-prone when the serum level of one electrolyte, potassium, becomes low. Serum electrolytes should be monitored at regular intervals throughout the operative and postoperative periods.

The amount of postoperative cardiac failure, not strangely, correlates with the amount of preoperative cardiac failure caused by the disease process. Preoperative left ventricular performance can be assessed by a cine-ventriculogram, in which a radiopaque contrast medium is injected into the left ventricle and recorded on 35mm movie film (Figures 13.6 and 13.7). If there is considerable ventricular dysfunction, the heart team must take precautions to ensure adequate myocardial protection during interruptions in coronary blood flow, such as aortic cross-clamping.

During the ventriculogram, a method may be used to measure the amount of cardiac dysfunction. This method measures the ventricular volume. The difference in the amount of blood remaining in the ventricle during systole, as opposed to the amount of blood remaining in the ventricle during diastole is the amount of blood "ejected" with each heartbeat (or the stroke volume). The ratio of stroke volume to end-diastolic volume is called "the ejection fraction." The ejection fraction is a sensitive index of cardiac performance. Normal ejection fractions are approximately 0.67. With cardiac failure, the ejection fraction decreases.

Postoperative Hemorrhage

The human body has a remarkable ability to "auto-regulate" (compensate) for changes in blood volume. For example, a blood donor's body auto-regulates the blood volume to allow for the sudden loss of a unit of blood. In a serious trauma case, the effects of a sudden drop in blood

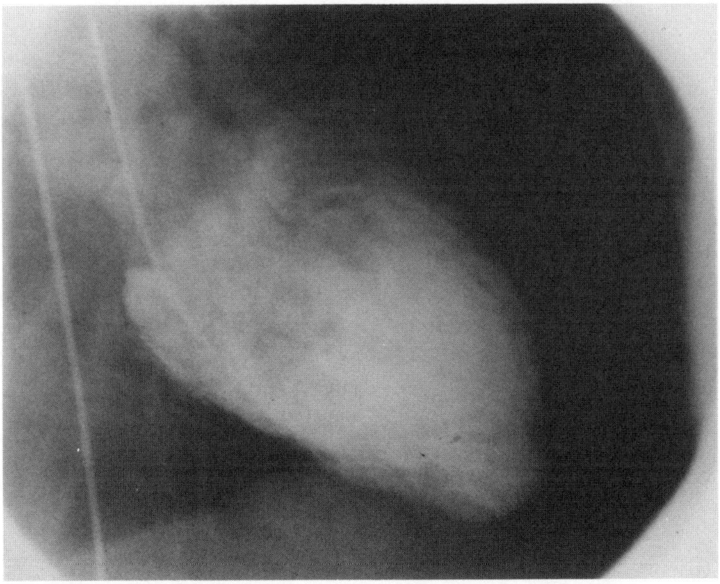

Figure 13.6 Ventricular injection of radiopaque contrast medium during diastole. Normal left ventriculogram, 30° right anterior oblique, maximum diastole. (Figures 13.6 and 13.7 courtesy of E. Lawrence Ganter, M.D. (retired), Phoenix, Arizona.)

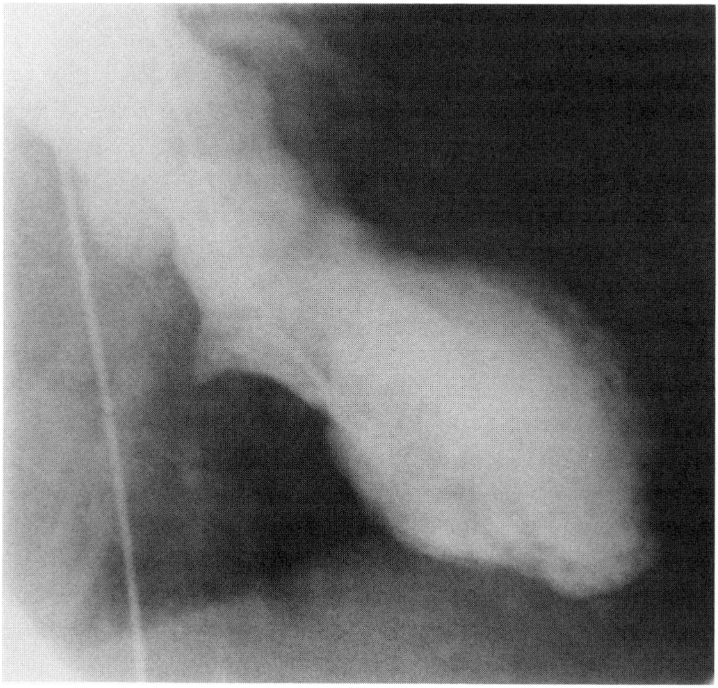

Figure 13.7 Ventricular injection of radiopaque contrast medium during systole. Normal left ventriculogram, 30° right anterior oblique, maximum systole.

volume are compensated by a "pooling" of blood in the vital organs (core circulation) and a decrease in circulation to the peripheral organs (skin and muscle tissue). During cardiopulmonary bypass, blood volume shifts are extensive. For example, at the beginning of bypass, the patient's blood is diluted by the priming fluid that is used to fill the heart-lung machine. The amount of this kind of dilution is commonly measured by the "mixed hematocrit." (You may remember that hematocrit is the laboratory process used to measure the cellular volume of a blood sample.) The mixed hematocrit reflects the dilutional effect caused by the priming fluid-blood mixture. The dilutional effect upon the formed elements of the blood diminishes the efficiency of blood cell physiology. The red cells have a diminished oxygen-carrying capacity (anemia). Dilution of the platelets reduces the blood's clotting ability. The dilution of the white cells results in their decreased ability to fight bacteria. Dilutional effects, destruction of the formed elements of the blood, and destruction of the plasma proteins all lead to alterations in the postoperative hematological state of the patient. Thus, it is important to closely monitor hematological values in the postoperative period. Packed red blood cells may be administered to replace the dilution of red blood cells. Fresh frozen plasma may be administered to replace the lost clotting elements normally found in the plasma. Occasionally, platelets are also administered to help restore normal coagulation.

Inadequate postoperative blood volume (hypovolemia) is characterized by low cardiac output and hypotension. Decreased tissue perfusion leads to metabolic acidosis, which further decreases the heart's ability to pump blood. This circular and sometimes deadly path is called "hypovolemic shock." Normal blood volume may be restored by the administration of whole blood or blood products and intravenous solutions.

Pulmonary Failure

One common respiratory problem following open

heart surgery is decreased ventilation. This condition may be a side effect of the anesthesia, the surgery itself (the process of entering the thoracic cavity is in itself abnormal, requiring positive pressure ventilation), or the pain resulting from the surgical incision. Also, drugs (such as curare and anectine) are commonly given to cause a temporary paralysis of the thoracic musculature. These drugs require time to lose their effect.

Another complication is respiratory failure. It is usually caused by the pre-existing disease, such as chronic obstructive pulmonary disease (asthma, emphysema, chronic bronchitis, bronchiectasis). Respiratory failure may also be caused by pulmonary emboli, characterized by a sudden onset of dyspnea or unexplained chest pain.

Yet another complication involving the respiratory system is pulmonary edema, secondary to cardiac failure. Symptoms include dyspnea caused by decreased oxygen tension and elevated carbon dioxide tension.

Any of these respiratory postoperative complications may be treated by prolonged endotracheal intubation and supported by means of mechanical ventilation.

Renal Failure

Renal complications following open heart surgery are largely caused by underlying renal disease, such as nephritis and tubular necrosis. However, a prolonged hypotensive episode in the operating room may cause acute renal failure by producing renal ischemia. Symptoms include decreased urinary output, an elevated potassium level, and an elevated BUN.

Infection

Several kinds of infection may complicate postoperative recovery from open heart surgery. Among them are atelectasis, pulmonary infection, urinary tract infection, and wound infection. While the incidence of postoperative infection is no higher in open heart surgery than in any other major surgery, the consequences may be dramatically more serious because of the kind of underlying disease that the patient has. Generally, a broad spectrum antibiotic is given pre-operatively to reduce the risk of infection.

If significant blood trauma has occurred from the use of the heart lung machine, the complement activation system may be impaired (see Chapter Twelve).

Footnotes

[1]E. Converse Pierce II, M.D., *Extracorporeal Circulation For Open Heart Surgery* (Springfield, Illinois: Charles C. Thomas, 1969), pp. 3 and 4.

DESIRES, NEEDS, & CONCLUSIONS

CHAPTER FOURTEEN

No one has a crystal ball with which to gaze into the future. However, by observing trends in one's field of study, one may predict the high probability of some events.

Le Gallois, as we mentioned at the beginning of this book, predicted artificial circulation some one hundred and forty years before its actual realization. Reflecting on Monsieur Le Gallois' prediction, we realize that perhaps predictions for the future are at some point manifested as desires for the future. It seems a universal truth that Man's desires and needs have lead the way to his most useful inventions. It was the desire of M. Le Gallois to preserve a mammalian organism by finding a way to provide artificially oxygenated blood to the organism in a manner similar to the way the natural heart functions that ultimately led in 1953 to Dr. Gibbons' use of a heart-lung machine to repair a atrial-septal defect in the heart of a young girl.

Some critics of medical research question the value of such research to society, especially when considered in light of the tremendous expenditures of money which sometimes needs to be made in order to conduct such research. When Benjamin Franklin, one of America's great statesmen, inventors, and philosophers, was questioned about the value of basic research, he answered with a question: "What is the use of a newborn baby?" The value of any basic research advancement is its value for the future.

Other critics may fear the future or may fear change itself. For example, the Luddites, an early nineteenth century group of English workmen, organized themselves to destroy labor-saving machinery.

Basic research is of limited value unless it is adequately communicated by careful documentation and reportage and unless the knowledge that is acquired is ultimately put to use. What begins as a basic need is transformed into a usable technique or product by the efforts of a myriad of people. The basic scientist, the engineer, the writer, the medical manufacturer, the librarian, the technical sales representative, the perfusionist, and the physician are but a few in a long line of people responsible for a connection of events from inception to application.

With this philosophical background in mind, let's spend a few moments to express some of the desires for the future that we see in terms of the heart lung machine and related technologies.

Biocompatible Materials:

Whenever anyone contemplates the fabrication of a new extracorporeal apparatus, the choice of materials is always uppermost in their minds. New designs are often cast aside because of the lack of biocompatible materials.

A. Blood Contact Surfaces

It would certainly be desirable, for example, to fabricate a machine that has a perfect blood contact surface area—one that does not require anticoagulants to prevent clot formation. There has been considerable experimentation with compounds containing heparin to coat machine surfaces that come in contact with the blood. Unfortunately, surface-coating compounds can be "washed" away and thereby lose their effectiveness. Too, the residual effect of the "washed off" compound may be undesirable.

Some polyurethanes are presently used in artificial heart designs. These plastics have relatively antithrombotic surfaces. However, such compounds are very expensive, and at present are rarely used for short term applications in heart lung machines.

Even the most biocompatible materials known to man fall far short of perfection. The "perfect" material, of course, is the human endothelium, which lines the entire natural circulatory system. Attempts are underway by a number of scientists to culture endothelial linings onto the surface of synthetic materials and then to use these cultured surfaces to fabricate intracorporeal and extracorporeal blood-handling devices, such as artificial hearts and heart lung machines.

B. Defoaming Agents

For years, defoaming agents have been used to coat surfaces in order to decrease the surface tension of the blood, causing the bubbles which come in contact with those surfaces to burst. These agents are used primarily in the fabrication of bubble-type artificial lungs (see Chapter Five). These defoaming agents can also be gradually washed from the surface, thus losing their effectiveness and possibly causing embolization. An ideal material is needed that can decrease the surface tension of bubbles without being washed off.

C. Roller Blood Pump Tubing

Although no one can discount its simplicity and reliability, the DeBakey roller-type blood pump (patented in 1937) is not an ideal pump. A number of investigators have shown that roller-type pumps spall (chip, flake) material from their lumenal surfaces. Spalled particles of tubing can lodge in the blood vessels and cause embolization. However, the amount of lumenal spallation seems acceptable for the short amount of time that patients are on cardiopulmonary bypass, and inline filters remove most of these particles. An ideal pump would not generate particulate material. However, materials technology may solve the problem of spallation. For example, present tubing materials are usually polyvinylchloride or silicone. Some experiments have been made with polyurethane tubing which showed minimal spallation.

Blood Pumps:

An ideal blood pump would produce a pulsatile flow pattern. A number of pulsatile pumps have been designed and produced. However, the theoretical advantage of pulsatile flow has not outweighed the practical disadvantages imposed by the large bore cannulas which must be used in order to deliver a physiologically acceptable pulsatile flow.

An ideal blood pump would be easily calibrated and would deliver its flow over a wide range of outlet resistances. Present day roller-type pumps do meet these criteria. Centrifugal-type pumps, on the other hand, are not readily calibrated and do not deliver a constant flow with varying outlet resistances.

An ideal blood pumping system would be incapable of pumping air. The best pumping system presently available in this respect is the centrifugal-type pump. Once blood has been displaced by air in the centrifugal-type blood pump housing, the pump will no longer pump liquid—it must be primed again. This process acts as a safety mechanism in the event air enters the pump housing.

The ideal blood pumping system should not create suction on its inlet side. One solution has been designed that was named the "perfusion-loop" by its inventors (Figure 14.1). The perfusion-loop is a double-walled tube. The inner wall or inner tube is very thin and collapsible. The outer wall or tube is more like a conventional kind of roller-type blood pump tubing. This device is inserted into a conventional roller-type blood pump housing. If the inlet pressure is less than zero, the inner tube collapses, thus preventing the pump from pumping fluids (both liquids and gases). This type of pump can be set up in systems that will not pump air.

Oxygenation Systems:

The trend in artificial blood oxygenation systems is toward membrane-type artificial lungs and away from bubble-type artificial lungs. Gas exchange takes place across a permeable membrane in the membrane-type lung, thus avoiding any direct blood-gas interface (see Chapter Five). As a result, much of the blood trauma created in a bubble-type oxygenator is avoided. This is not to say that the bubble-type oxygenator does not have its proponents, nor does it mean that the bubble-type oxygenator will be summarily replaced. It has had the reputation of the "work horse" of gas exchange devices for a number of years. It is a simple, cost effective, and versatile device. Replacement of bubble-type artificial lungs by membrane-type artificial lungs will be a slow process.

Sometime in the far off but foreseeable future, mo-

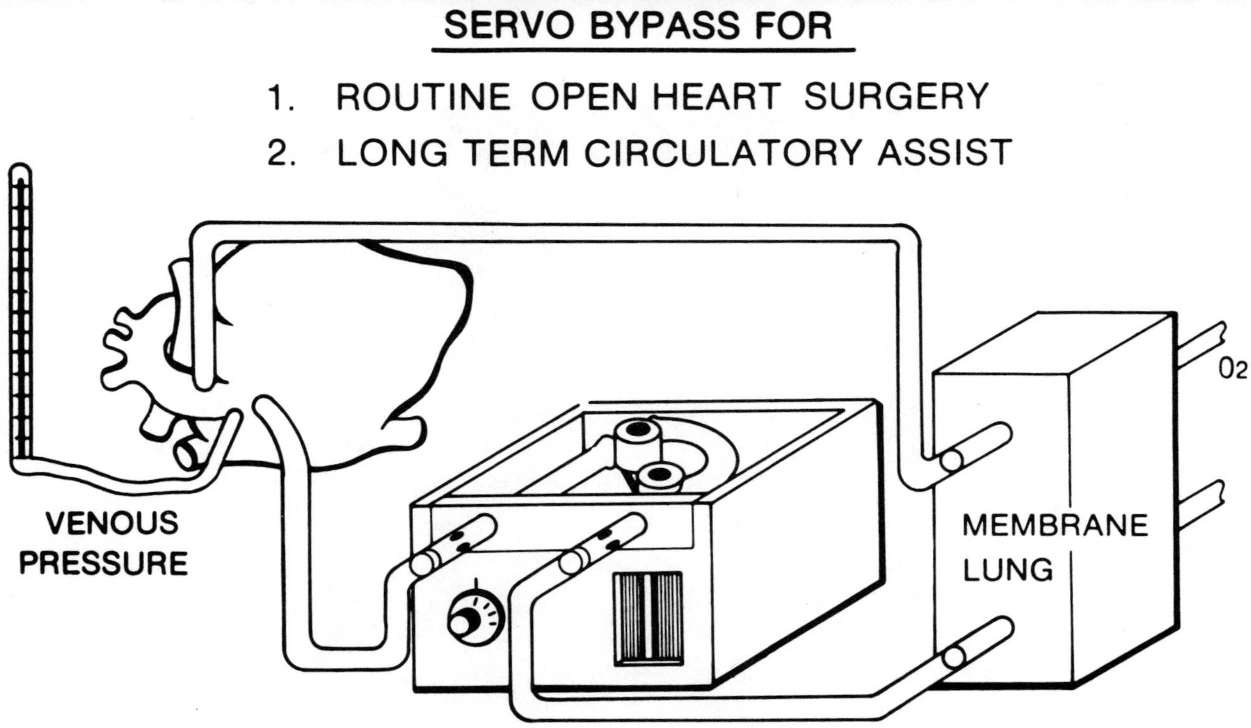

Figure 14.1 The perfusion loop does not create suction at its inlet side.

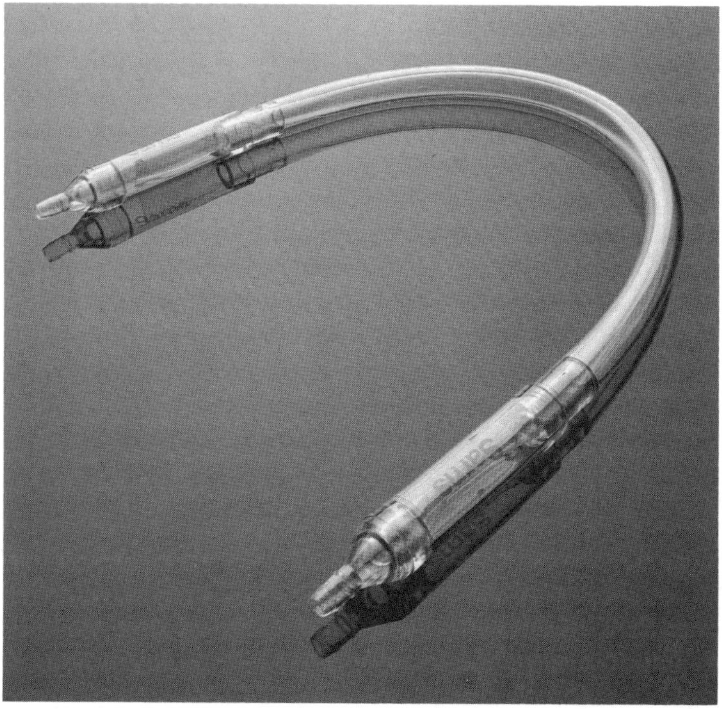

Figure 14.2 The Safety Loop (perfusion loop) is designed to protect the heart from damaging pressures that can be generated in the venting system during cardiopulmonary bypass surgery. (Courtesy of Sarns, 3M Healthcare, Ann Arbor, Michigan.)

bile, wearable artificial lungs may be used in the treatment of chronic obstructive pulmonary diseases such as emphysema. Thought has also been given to a totally implantable artificial lung.

Monitoring Systems:

Continuous monitoring of a number of physiological parameters has been available for many years. Arterial and venous pressure is continuously measured and displayed by most open-heart surgical teams. It is becoming more common for open-heart teams to continuously monitor and display blood gas parameters, such as pH, PCO_2, and PO_2 during the perfusion (Figure 14.3). This monitoring of blood gas parameters has been done extracorporeally up to the present time. Practical systems are now feasible which will measure and display blood gas parameters intracorporeally by means of indwelling catheters. Blood pressure can simultaneously be monitored by this method as well. In the foreseeable future, this same method (by means of indwelling catheters) will also measure electrolytes. Both kinds of systems are presently in the experimental stage.

Information Feedback Systems:

Some advanced computer monitoring systems are already in place to assist in the care of the open heart surgical patient. However, technologically speaking, we have only begun to row across a veritable ocean. We are limited only by the scope of our imaginations and the realities of our economies.

Computer monitoring systems have already been designed that continuously monitor and display many valuable physiological parameters—with the measurements displayed in hard number values rather than estimated values. Such systems measure and compare individual results with programmed normals with unceasing diligence. Alarms signal attending personnel if parameters stray out of optimal range (Figure 14.4).

Heart lung machines will soon be equipped with

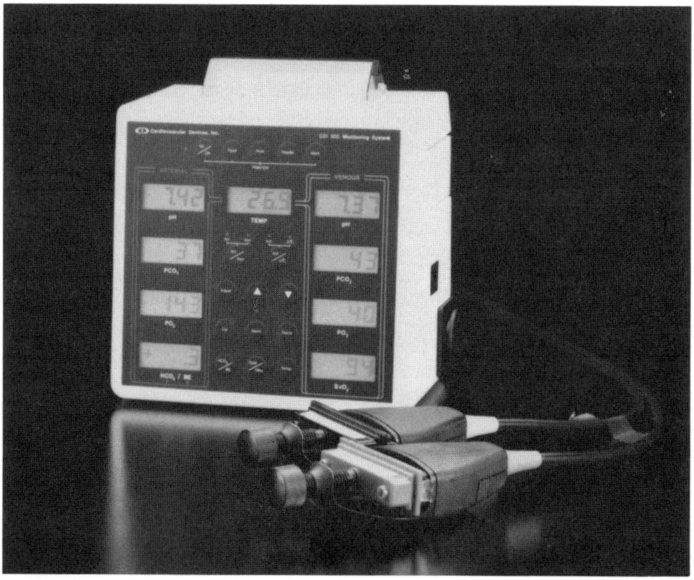

Figure 14.3 Continous blood gas monitoring system. (Courtesy CDI, 3M Healthcare, Irvine, California.)

automatic feedback systems that will measure and adjust various temperatures, acid-base parameters, and blood flow rates (Figure 14.8). In our opinion, perfusionists should not form Luddite groups to prevent such automation. We feel that such systems will enhance the professional role of the perfusionist rather than detract from it. Perfusionists will not only have to know how to operate the automated systems, they will also have to know how to override these systems and to operate the machines manually.

Blood Substitutes and Blood Recovery Systems:

Autotransfusion systems are technologically feasible that can recover nearly all of the blood lost during the course of an open heart operation. Presently, systems are in use that can recover chest tube drainage and reuse the blood (Figure 14.10). Blood has become an increasingly valuable resource. Future needs will focus upon blood conservation and improved blood recovery systems.

There was intense interest a few years ago in "artificial blood," and some countries, such as Japan, are presently using it. However, the fluorocarbons that compose artificial blood remains as a residue in the body. Although these compounds are biologically inert for the short term, the long term effects of the compounds are not well understood. Until the long term effects of residual fluorocarbon have been properly assessed, their use will be limited. The need for a reliable blood substitute continues because of the increase of blood-related diseases and the high cost and dwindling supply of donor blood.

Circulatory Assist and Cardiac Replacement:

The future of circulatory assist is very dependent, as are other extracorporeal applications, upon further advancements in material technology. The most limiting component for successful long term circulatory assistance has been the necessity for systemic heparinization. With recent successes in cardiac transplantation, the current trend is to apply circulatory assist or to use artificial heart replacement as an

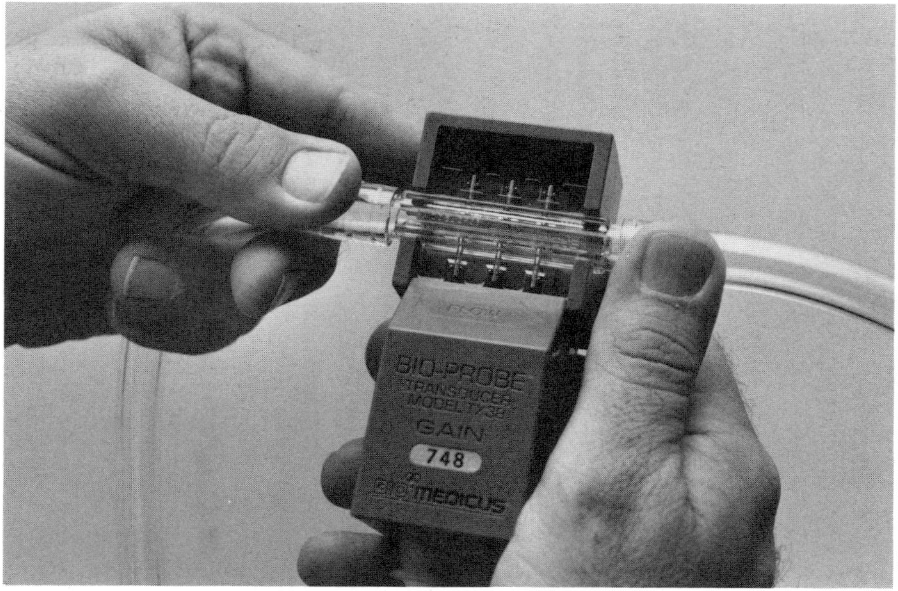

Figure 14.4 Disposable blood flow probe. The blood flow signal can be fed into a computer. (Courtesy of Biomedicus, Minnetonka, Minnesota.)

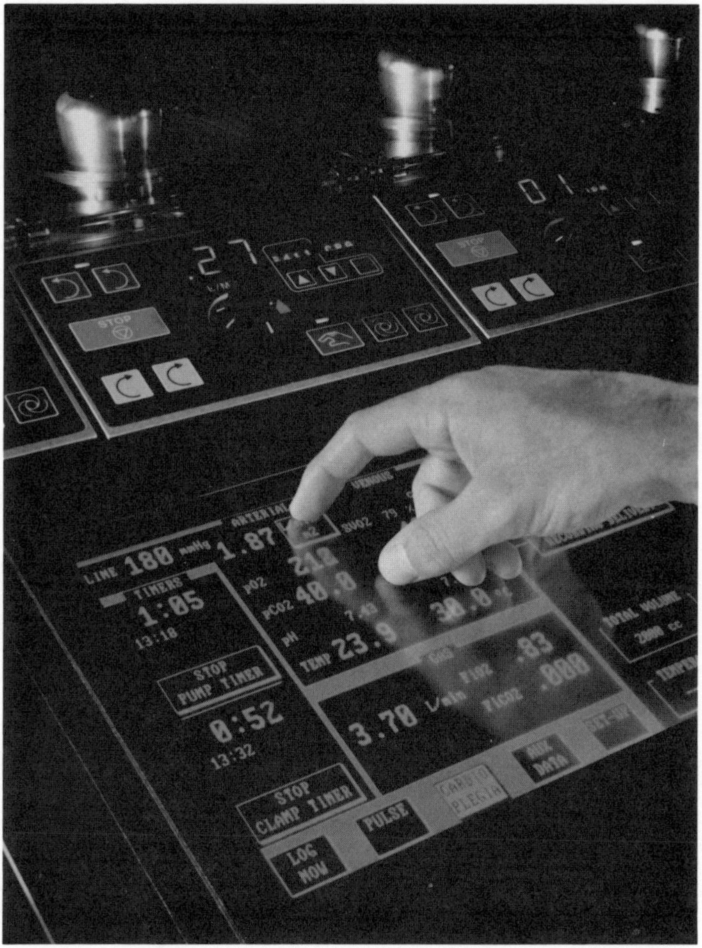

Figure 14.5 Touch screen control for a heart-lung machine. (Courtesy of Sarns, 3M Healthcare, Ann Arbor, Michigan.)

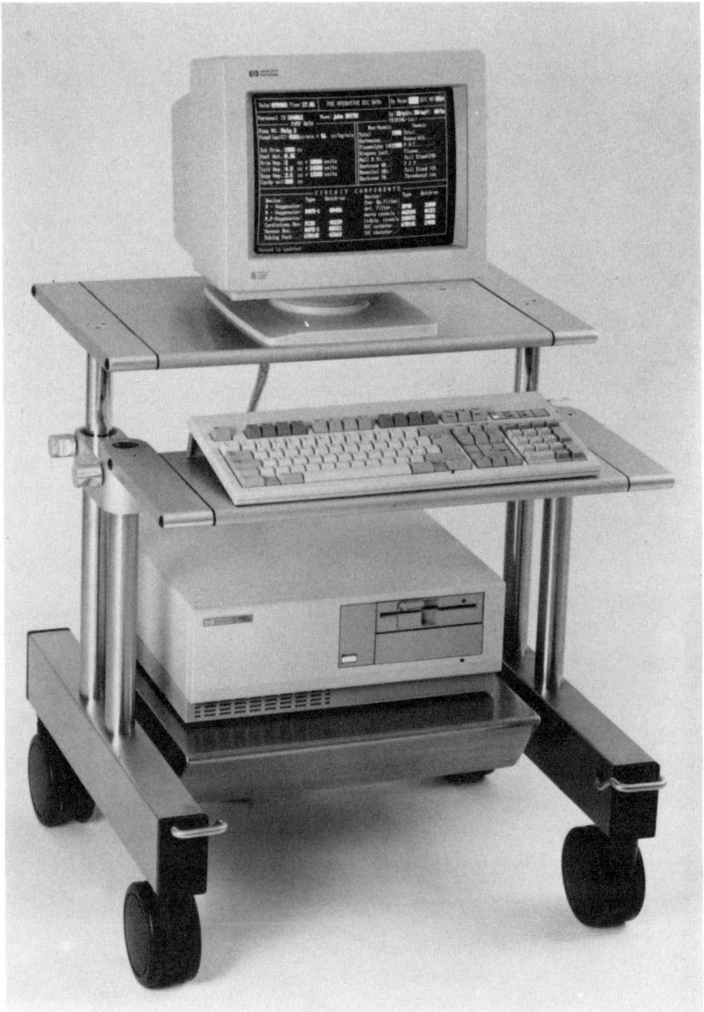

Figure 14.6 This computer program for extracorporeal circulation has been developed for use with a heart-lung machine and an IBM® or compatible computer. (Courtesy of Vitalcor, Inc. (Polystan), Westmont, Illinois.)

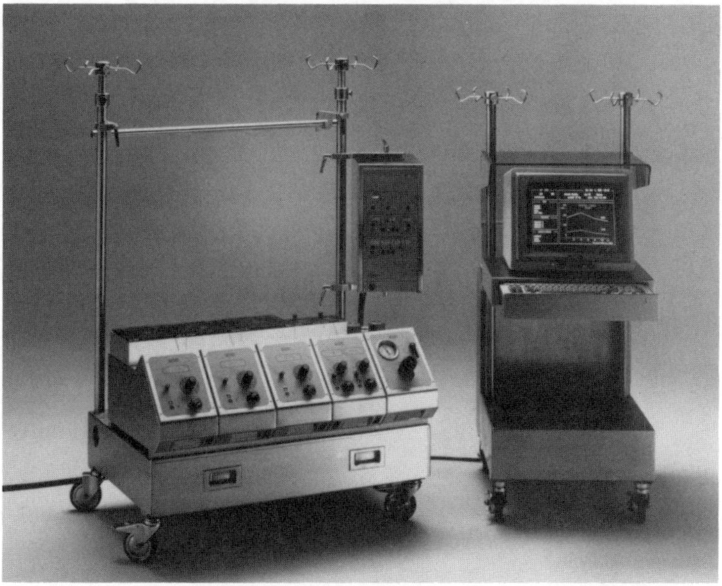

Figure 14.7 A modular heart-lung system consisting of roller pumps and monitoring-controlling devices, including a computerized perfusion data management program. (Courtesy of Shiley, Inc., Irvine, California.)

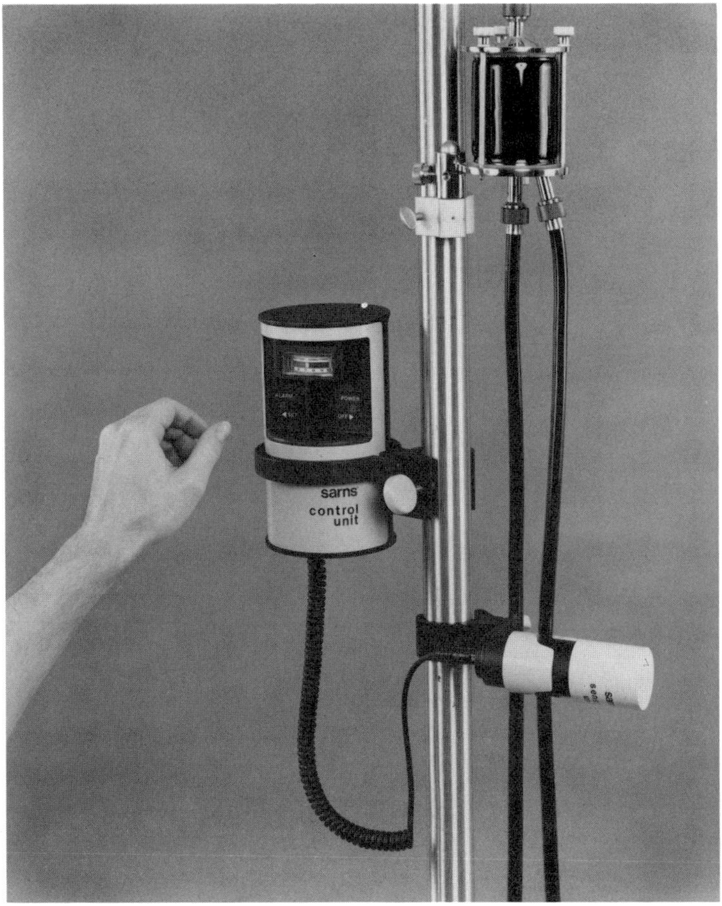

Figure 14.8 Automatic shut-off device for heart-lung machine. If air passes through the sensor, the machine will shut off instantaneously. (Courtesy of Sarns, 3M Healthcare, Ann Arbor, Michigan.)

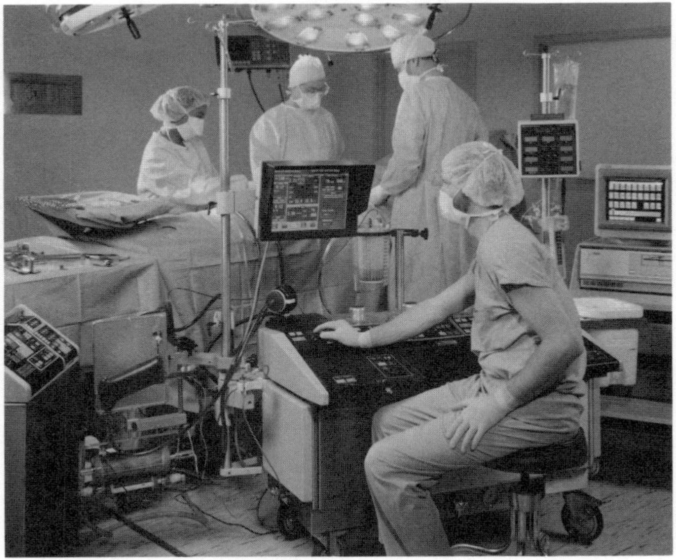

Figure 14.9 A computer-controlled open heart simulator helps train perfusionists to use new equipment without risk to a patient. (Courtesy of Sarns, 3M Healthcare, Ann Arbor, Michigan.)

interim measure until a donor heart can be found and transplanted. The problem, of course, is the shortage of donor organs. Society must be prepared, through education, to donate voluntarily the organs of those who can no longer use them. Extracorporeal circulatory assist devices are presently of limited value for long term circulatory support.

Permanent Artificial Cardiac Replacement:

Although the problems of cardiac replacement with a total artificial heart have been widely publicized, the time is not far off that successful replacement of the human heart with a mechanical heart will be technologically practical. Present devices are but mere forerunners of the modern era of artificial hearts.

The authors feel that society is technologically impatient. We are accustomed to high speed technological development. The artificial heart is technologically at the corresponding point in time of the Wright brothers' airplane. At that time, the public questioned the value of a machine that could fly only 120 feet. Twenty-four years later, Lindbergh flew from New York to Paris. Sixty-six years after the Wright brothers' attempts, man first set foot on the moon. Within the span of a lifetime, the practicality of flight advanced from 120 feet to 221,900 miles.

The analogy has been made that the quality of life of a artificial heart recipient linked to a heart-driver console is as acceptable as the quality of life of a paraplegic linked to a wheelchair. However, the number of strokes associated with the present implantation of total artificial hearts is not acceptable as a quality of life issue. We hope that the mechanical hearts of the future will eliminate this problem.

A major stumbling block to further development of the total artificial heart is inadequate money to finance research expenditures. The projected costs are enormous for each individual use. Some feel that we cannot afford to apply the technology once it is perfected. Others feel that the money should not be spent on "old people" who have a limited lifespan and limited value to society. Whatever the economic, social, and moral principles involved, we feel that we can ill afford not to continue to develop the artificial heart. The number of people who can benefit from this technology is extremely high. There are thousands of relatively young people who die each year from myocardial infarctions and from cardiac failure.

Alternatives to Open Heart Surgery:

As an ultimate goal, prevention of a disease always takes priority over the treatment of a disease. In terms of heart disease, we have seen the value of preventative measures in recent years. Rheumatic heart disease, a significant cause of valvular heart disease, can be treated effectively with antibiotics, thereby preventing valvular stenosis and regurgitation. Coronary artery disease (although still the leading cause of death in this country) is now on the decline. Causative factors such as diet, lack of exercise, and cigarette smoking have been identified and publicized. The public seems to be slowly responding to the need to assume responsibility for its own health care.

Until the goal of prevention is accomplished, however, we must depend on new and better treatments for heart disease. For example, another alternative to open heart surgery has been the increased use of coronary angioplasty. At the time of cardiac catheterization, a balloon catheter is inserted into a coronary artery and inflated with saline. Atherosclerotic plaque is compressed against the wall of the diseased artery, thus enlarging its lumen and improving blood flow to the heart muscle. Controversy about the long term benefit of the procedure still continues, but it has been proven that the procedure has value for a select group of patients.

Experimental studies are underway on other therapies for the treatment of coronary artery disease. Catheters have been developed which can direct a laser light beam that "vaporizes" plaque in the coronary arteries. A "roto-rooter" catheter is under development that can remove the plaque by means of a tiny rotating blade. The particles of plaque can

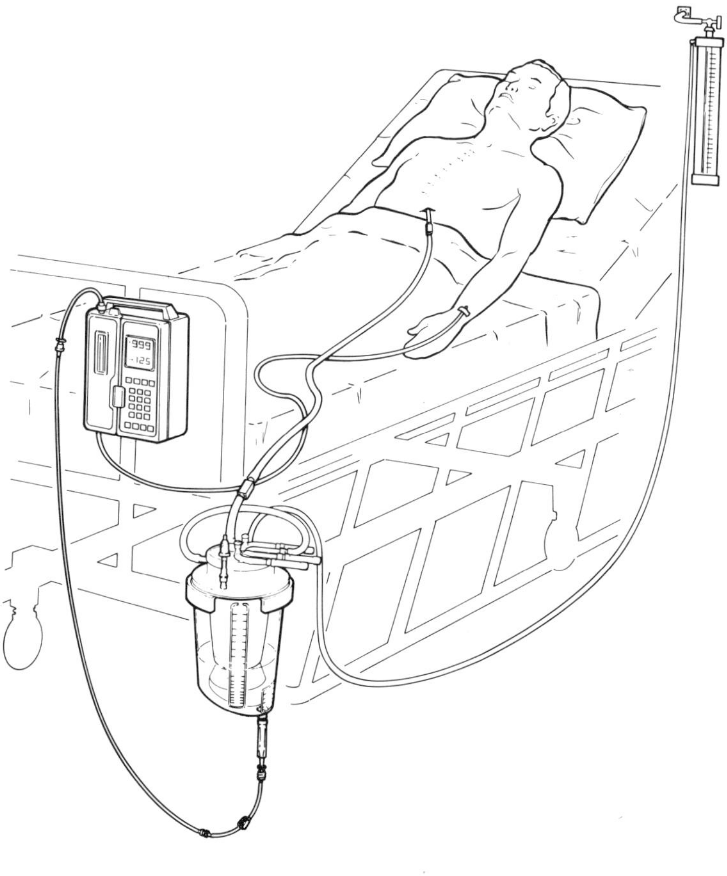

Figure 14.10 Blood recovery system designed to recover chest tube drainage of postoperative patients. (Courtesy of Baxter Healthcare Corporation, Bentley Laboratories Division, Irvine, California.)

then be removed by aspiration. The technique is similar to the phacoemulsification procedure that is used by ophthalmologists in the extracapsular removal of cataractal lenses.

Conclusion:

It should be noted here that by the time this book is printed, some of the desires and needs for improved equipment and techniques that we have mentioned may have already resulted in their invention or production. The linkages of ideas that result from increased scientific knowledge produce rapid changes in technology. It is our hope that you, the readers of this book, will play an important role in the solution of the problems necessary to make many of these desires and needs become reality.

Appendix

Normal Values Acid-Base Chemistry of Whole Blood

Arterial Blood	
pH	7.38-7.44
PCO2	35-40 mm Hg
PO_2	95-100 mmHg
O_2 SAT	94-100%
CO_2 Content	19-24 mM/L
B.E.	-2.5 to +2.5

Venous Blood	
pH	7.36-7.41
PCO_2	40-45 mm HG
CO_2 Content	22-26 mM/L
B.E.	-2.5 to +2.5

Normal Values
Hematology

Activated Clotting Time **	Approx. 100-120 Sec. (whole blood).
Blood Volume	Male: 69 ml/Kg Female: 65 ml/Kg
Fibrinogen	200-400 mg/dl (plasma)
Hematocrit	Male: 40-54% Female: 38-47%
Hemoglobin	Male: 13.5-18 gm/dl Female: 12.0-16 gm/dl
Partial Thromboplastin Time	60-70 Seconds
Platelet Count	150,000-400,000/ul
Plasma Volume	Male: 39 ml/Kg Female: 40 ml/Kg
Prothrombin Time	12-14 seconds
Red Cell Count	Male: 4.6-6.2 X 10^6/ul Female: 4.2-5.4 X 10^6/ul
Viscosity	1.4-1.8 Times Water
White Cell Count	4,500-11,000/ul

** Values may vary with different techniques

Normal Values
Chemistry of Blood

Bicarbonate	21-28 mM/L (plasma)
Calcium	9.0-10.6 mg/dl (serum)
Chloride	95-103 mEq/L (serum)
Cholesterol	150-250 mg/dl (serum)
Creatine	Male: 0.2-0.6 mg/dl Female: 0.6-1.0 mg/dl (serum)
Fibrinogen	200-400 mg/dl (plasma)
Glucose, fasting	70-110 mg/dl (serum)
Plasma Hemoglobin	0.5-5.0 mg/dl (serum or plasma)
Hemoglobin	Male: 13.5-18.0 gm/dl Female: 12.0-16.0 gm/dl (blood)
Magnesium	1.5-2.5 mEq/L (serum)
Osmolality	280-295 mOsm/L (serum)
Potassium	3.8-5.0 mEq/L (plasma)
Sodium	136-142 mEq/L (plasma)
Triglycerides	10-190 mg/dl (serum)
Urea Nitrogen	8-18 mg/dl (serum)

Hemodynamic Parameters

Parameter	Definition	Normal Values
Blood Flow Rate (ml/min) Body Wt. (Kg) **ml/min/Kg=** $\frac{CO}{Wt}$	Total Blood Flow Rate (CO) indexed to body weight	Opinions vary about "adequate blood flow rate." Range: 40-100 ml/min/Kg
Arterial Blood Pressure (BPA)	Pressure exerted by blood on arterial walls.	Varies with age. Adult: 130/70 mm Hg
Central Venous Pressure (CVP)	Pressure of blood within the central venous system (in or near the vena cavae.)	4-10 mm Hg Increases with cardiac failure
Systemic Vascular Resistance (SVR) $SVR = \frac{BPA-CVP}{CO} \times 80$ (Blood pressures are expressed as means.)	Resistance to blood flow in the systemic circulation or opposition to blood flow throughout the systemic circulation.	Adult: 900-1500 dyne-sec/cm $^{-5}$

Hemodynamic Parameters

Parameter	Definition	Normal Values
Cardiac Output (CO) **CO = HR X SV**	Total blood flow rate or quantity of blood ejected by the heart each minute	Varies with body size. Adult: 4-8 L/min
Heart Rate (HR)	Number of times the heart beats	Adult: 60-100 bpm
Stroke Volume (SV) $SV = \frac{CO}{HR}$	Volume of blood ejected by the heart with each beat	Adult: 60-130 ml/beat
Body Surface Area (BSA) $BSA = 71.84 \times Wt.^{.425} \times Ht.^{.725}$ Wt = Weight (Kg) Ht. = Height (cm) BSA = Body Surface Area (M^2)	Surface area of the body as estimated by the DuBois Formula.	Varies with body size. Example: Wt. = 70 Kg Ht. = 175 cm BSA = 1.84 M^2
Cardiac Index (CI) $CI = \frac{CO}{BSA}$ also **CO = CI X BSA**	Cardiac Index is an adjustment of cardiac output for body size (BSA). It is used by some perfusionists as a method of calculating blood flow rate during cardiovascular perfusion.	Varies with body size. Adult: 2.5-3.1 L/min/m^2

GENERAL REFERENCES AND SUGGESTED READING

Berger, E.C. *The Physiology of Adequate Perfusion*. St. Louis: The C.V. Mosby Company, 1979.

Braunwald, E.A., ed. *Heart Disease*. Philadelphia: W.B. Saunders Company, 1980.

Brecher, G.A., and P.M. Galletti. *Heart-Lung Bypass*. New York: Grune & Statton, Inc., 1956.

Davenport, H. *The ABC of Acid-Base Chemistry*. Chicago: The University of Chicago Press, 1974.

Ionescu, M.I., ed. *Techniques in Extracorporeal Circulation*. Second Edition. London: Butterworths, 1981.

Kennedy, J.H. *Support of the Failing Circulation*. Springfield: Charles C. Thomas Publishing, 1967.

Kirklin, J.W., and B.G. Barrett-Boyles. *Cardiac Surgery*. New York: John Wiley & Sons, 1986.

Petz, L.D., and S.N. Swisher, eds. *Clinical Practice of Blood Transfusion*. New York: Churchill Livingstone, Inc., 1981.

Pierce, E.C. *Extracorporeal Circulation for Open Heart Surgery*. Springfield: Charles C. Thomas, 1969.

Quail, S. *Comprehensive Intra-Aortic Balloon Pumping*. St. Louis: The C.V. Mosby Company, 1984.

Reed, C.C., M. Kurusz, and A. E. Lawrence. *Safety and Techniques in Perfusion*. Stafford, Texas: Quali-Med Inc., 1988.

Reed, C.C., and T. Stafford. *Cardiopulmonary Bypass*. Second Edition. Houston: Texas Medical Press, Inc., 1985.

Taylor, K.M. *Cardiopulmonary Bypass, Principles and Management*. Baltimore: Williams and Wilkins, 1986.

Williams, P.L., and R. Warwick, eds. *Gray's Anatomy*, 36th Edition. New York: Churchill Livingstone, 1980.

Index

About the Authors

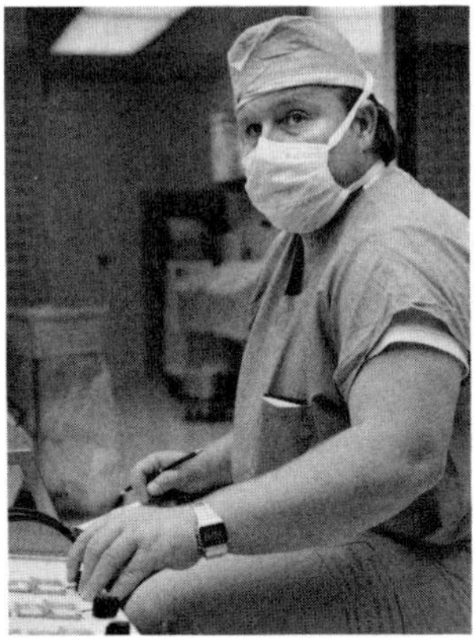

Jon W. Austin, C.C.P., is a full-time cardiovascular perfusionist. He attended Utah State University, majoring in physiology, then became a member of the research and clinical staff of the University of Utah. He is certified in the practice of clinical cardiovascular perfusion and has published many articles related to his field. Jon has several inventions with application to cardiovascular surgery that have been marketed. His most recent research interest has been with the artificial heart.

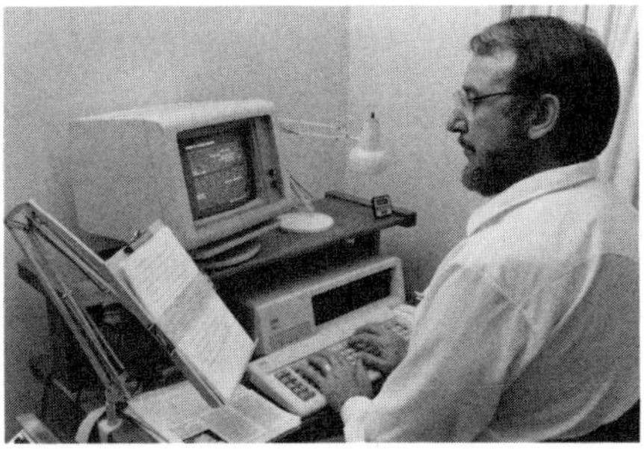

David L. Harner became a professional writer and publisher after spending ten years as Director of Education of a major Phoenix medical center. He attended Alexian Brothers Hospital School of Nursing in Chicago, Illinois; majored in English at Winona State University in Winona, Minnesota; and did graduate work in English at Northwestern University and California State University at Northridge. Dave has taught English at the high school and college level and has been involved with teaching and administering medical education programs for a variety of medical personnel. His specialty is writing medical and technical information in print and audiovisual media for lay audiences.